Navigating Life with
Amyotrophic Lateral Sclerosis

Lisa M. Shulman, MD, FAAN

Editor-in-Chief, *Neurology Now*™ Books Series
Fellow of the American Academy of Neurology
Professor of Neurology
The Eugenia Brin Professor in Parkinson's Disease and Movement Disorders
The Rosalyn Newman Distinguished Scholar in Parkinson's Disease
Director, University of Maryland PD & Movement Disorders Center
University of Maryland School of Medicine
Baltimore, MD

Other Titles in the *Neurology Now*™ Books Series

Navigating Life with Parkinson's Disease
Sortirios A. Parashos, MD, PhD; Rose Wichmann, PT; and Todd Melby

Navigating Life with a Brain Tumor
Lynne P. Taylor, MD, FAAN; Alyx B. Porter Umphrey, MD; and Diane Richard

Navigating the Complexities of Stroke
Louis R. Caplan, MD, FAAN

Navigating Life with Multiple Sclerosis
Kathleen Costello, MS, ANP-BC, MSCN; Ben W. Thrower, MD;
and Barbara S. Giesser, MD

Navigating Life with Epilepsy
David C. Spencer, MD, FAAN

Navigating Life with Amyotrophic Lateral Sclerosis

Mark B. Bromberg, MD, PhD, FAAN

Department of Neurology
University of Utah
Salt Lake City, Utah

Diane Banks Bromberg, JD

Fabian VanCott
Salt Lake City, Utah

OXFORD
UNIVERSITY PRESS

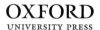

OXFORD
UNIVERSITY PRESS

Oxford University Press is a department of the University of Oxford. It furthers the University's objective of excellence in research, scholarship, and education by publishing worldwide. Oxford is a registered trade mark of Oxford University Press in the UK and certain other countries.

Published in the United States of America by Oxford University Press
198 Madison Avenue, New York, NY 10016, United States of America.

Library of Congress Cataloging-in-Publication Data
Names: Bromberg, M. B. (Mark B.), author. | Banks-Bromberg, Diane, author.
Title: Navigating life with ALS / by Mark B. Bromberg, MD, FAAN, Department of Neurology, University of Utah, Salt Lake City, UT,
Diane Banks-Bromberg, JD, Fabian Vancott, Salt Lake City, UT.
Description: New York, NY : American Academy of Neurology/Oxford University Press, [2017] | Includes index.
Identifiers: LCCN 2016036224 | ISBN 9780190241629 (alk. paper)
Subjects: LCSH: Amyotrophic lateral sclerosis—Popular works.
Classification: LCC RC406.A24 B76 2017 | DDC 616.8/39—dc23
LC record available at https://lccn.loc.gov/2016036224

This material is not intended to be, and should not be considered, a substitute for medical or other professional advice. Treatment for the conditions described in this material is highly dependent on the individual circumstances. And, while this material is designed to offer accurate information with respect to the subject matter covered and to be current as of the time it was written, research and knowledge about medical and health issues is constantly evolving and dose schedules for medications are being revised continually, with new side effects recognized and accounted for regularly. Readers must therefore always check the product information and clinical procedures with the most up-to-date published product information and data sheets provided by the manufacturers and the most recent codes of conduct and safety regulation. The publisher and the authors make no representations or warranties to readers, express or implied, as to the accuracy or completeness of this material. Without limiting the foregoing, the publisher and the authors make no representations or warranties as to the accuracy or efficacy of the drug dosages mentioned in the material. The authors and the publisher do not accept, and expressly disclaim, any responsibility for any liability, loss or risk that may be claimed or incurred as a consequence of the use and/or application of any of the contents of this material.

1 3 5 7 9 8 6 4 2
Printed by Sheridan Books, Inc., United States of America

We dedicate this book to Lois F. Hall and her husband, Ray A. Hall, parents of Diane Banks Bromberg. Lois rose to the challenges of ALS and lived her life enthusiastically until her passing. She participated in a drug trial that she hoped would shed light on this disease for the benefit of future patients. Ray unselfishly dedicated himself to helping Lois through her illness in every way possible.

CONTENTS

ABOUT THE AAN'S *NEUROLOGY NOW*™ BOOKS SERIES

Here is a question for you:

If you know more about your neurologic condition, will you do better than if you know less?

Well, not simply optimism but hard data show that individuals who are more knowledgeable about their medical conditions *do have better outcomes*. So learning about your neurologic condition plays an important role in doing the very best you can. The main purpose of both the *Neurology Now*™ Books series and *Neurology Now* magazine from the American Academy of Neurology (AAN) and the American Brain Foundation (ABF) is to focus on the needs of people with neurologic disorders. Our goal is to view neurologic issues through the eyes of people with neurologic problems, in order to understand and respond to their practical day-to-day needs.

So, you are probably saying, *"Of course, knowledge is a good thing, but how can it change the course of my disease?"* Well, healthcare is really a two-way street. After you have had a stroke, you need to find a knowledgeable and trusted neurologist; however, no physician can overcome the obstacle of working with inaccurate or incomplete information. Your physician is working to navigate the clues you provide in your own words combined with the clues from their neurologic examination, in order to arrive at an accurate diagnosis and respond to your individual needs. Many types of important clues exist, such as your description of your symptoms or your ability to identify how your neurologic condition affects your daily activities.

Poor patient-physician communication inevitably results in less-than-ideal outcomes. This problem is well described by the old adage, "garbage in, garbage out." The better you pin down and communicate your main problem(s), the more likely you are to walk out of your doctor's office with the plan that is right for you. Your neurologist is the expert in your disorder, but you and your family are the experts in "you." Physician decision-making is not a "one shoe fits all" enterprise, yet when accurate, individualized information is lacking, that's what it becomes.

Whether you are startled by hearing a new diagnosis or you come to this knowledge gradually, learning that you have a neurologic problem is jarring. Many neurologic disorders are chronic; you aren't simply adjusting to something new—you will need to deal with this disorder for the foreseeable future. In certain ways, life has changed. Now, there are two crucial "next steps": the first is finding good neurologic care for your problem, and the second is successfully adjusting to living with your condition. This second step depends on attaining knowledge of your condition, learning new skills to manage the condition, and finding the flexibility and resourcefulness to restore your quality of life. When successful, you regain your equilibrium and restore a sense of confidence and control that is the cornerstone of well-being.

When healthy adjustment does not occur following a new diagnosis, a sense of feeling out of control and overwhelmed often persists, and no doctor's prescription will adequately respond to this problem. Individuals who acquire good self-management skills are often able to recognize and understand new symptoms and take appropriate action. Conversely, those who are lacking in confidence may respond to the same symptom with a growing sense of anxiety and urgency. In the first case, "watchful waiting" or a call to the physician may result in resolution of the problem. In the second case, the uncertainty and anxiety often lead to multiple physician consultations, unnecessary new prescriptions, social withdrawal, or unwarranted hospitalization. Outcomes can be dramatically different depending on knowledge and preparedness.

Managing a neurologic disorder is new territory, and you should not be surprised that you need to be equipped with new information and a new skill set to effectively manage your condition. You will need to learn new words that describe both your symptoms and their treatment to communicate effectively with the members of your medical team. You will also need to learn how to gather accurate information about your condition when you need it and to avoid misinformation. Although all of your physicians document your progress in their medical records, keeping a personal journal about your neurologic condition will help you summarize and track all your medical information in one place. When you bring this journal with you as you go to see your physician, you will be able to provide more accurate information about your history and previous treatment. Your active and informed involvement in your care and decision-making results in a better quality of care and better outcomes.

Your neurologic condition is likely to pose new challenges in daily activities, including interactions in your family, your workplace, and your social and recreational activities. How can you best manage your symptoms or your medication dosing schedule in the context of your normal activities? When should you disclose your diagnosis to others? *Neurology Now* Books provide you with the background you need, including the experiences of others who have faced similar problems, to guide you through this unfamiliar terrain.

Our goal is to give you the resources you need to "take your doctor with you" when you confront these new challenges. We are committed to answering the questions and concerns of individuals living with neurologic disorders and their families in each volume of the *Neurology Now* Books series. We want you to be as prepared and confident as possible to participate with your doctors in your medical care. Much care is taken to develop each book with you in mind.

We include the most up-to-date, informative, and useful answers to the questions that most concern you—whether you find yourself in the unexpected role of patient or caregiver. Real-life experiences of patients and families are found throughout the text to illustrate important points. And feedback based on correspondence from *Neurology Now* magazine readers informs topics for new books and is integral to our quality improvement. These features are found in all books in the *Neurology Now* Books series so that you can expect the same quality and patient-centered approach in every volume.

I hope that you have arrived at a new understanding of why "knowledge is empowering" when it comes to your medical care and that *Neurology Now* Books will serve as an important foundation for the new skills you need to be effective in managing a neurologic condition.

Lisa M. Shulman, MD, FAAN
Editor-in-Chief, *Neurology Now*™ Books Series
Fellow of the American Academy of Neurology
Professor of Neurology
The Eugenia Brin Professor in Parkinson's Disease
and Movement Disorders
The Rosalyn Newman Distinguished Scholar
in Parkinson's Disease
Director, University of Maryland PD &
Movement Disorders Center
University of Maryland School of Medicine

FOREWORD

The past decade has seen a dramatic increase in the number of books about amyotrophic lateral sclerosis. Is this one truly needed? Yes, unequivocally. There is literature in which persons with ALS describe their experiences, and other literature in which medical personnel discuss ALS. The combined approach here is one that I am confident will be particularly meaningful to those living with ALS and their caregivers.

Physicians involved in the teaching and training of medical students and residents have long known that trainees learn much more effectively when presented with a combination of factual material and patient encounters. This book uses that approach by providing facts about ALS while concurrently permitting the reader to view ALS through the eyes of those with the disease and their loved ones.

The factual sections of the book are broad-ranging, covering virtually all aspects of ALS pathogenesis, presentation, evaluation, diagnosis, and management in a manner that is centered on what patients and their caregivers want to know or should know. The interweaving of patient and caregiver narratives throughout the book facilitates exploration of topics that are central to living with ALS but are rarely addressed. For example, the reader can feel the frustration that so many individuals with ALS feel as test after test is interpreted as "normal." At the same time, that reader also can find an explanation of the ALS evaluation that permits an understanding of why "normal" does not mean "no ALS." The sections on etiology and pathogenesis permit the authors to also tackle the "Why me?" question with which so many affected individuals and their caregivers struggle. I can easily imagine my patients and their caregivers thinking, "That's how I felt" or "That's what happened to me" as they read the narratives. Some sections are particularly poignant. "Living with ALS," for example, describes how individuals with ALS may change their perspectives on what is important to them for maintaining quality of life.

The authors bring together an uncommon combination of perspectives and skills. Dr. Mark Bromberg, a gifted and compassionate physician whom I have known for more than 25 years, has dedicated much of his professional career to the care of patients with ALS and to research centered around this devastating disease. His coauthor, Diane Banks Bromberg, has personally experienced the effects of ALS through her role as a caregiver for her mother. Their experiences frame the physician-caregiver-patient relationship so vital to those who face this disease's myriad physical, psychological, social, and existential consequences.

As a physician who has spent the past 25 years in ALS clinical care and research, I believe that Mark and Diane have done a tremendous service for our patients and their caregivers by producing this remarkable book, which is consistently informative and at various times inspiring, touching, heart-rending, and heartwarming. Mark states in the book's preface, "I try to put myself in the positions of the patient and caregiver." It is clear that he and Diane have written this book from that perspective, and in doing so have provided a much-needed resource to the ALS community.

Zachary Simmons, MD, FAAN
Fellow of the American Academy of Neurology
Professor of Neurology and Humanities
The Pennsylvania State University
Director, ALS Center
Penn State Hershey Medical Center

PREFACE

This is a book about ALS for patients with ALS, their caregivers, and other family members. ALS is perhaps the most challenging disease imaginable: researchers do not know what causes it or how to prevent it, no markedly effective treatments are available, and the disease is inexorably progressive. Not only does it affect the patient, but it has a life-changing impact on the primary caregiver and other members of the family.

I began working with patients with ALS early in my neurology career, and it has been my main clinical and research emphasis over the past 30 years. I established a special ALS clinic at the University of Michigan and then later established a second clinic at the University of Utah. I have participated in research efforts on using new techniques to make the diagnosis of ALS and am particularly interested in issues related to quality of life for people with the disease. I have also participated in many clinical drug trials related to ALS in the hope of better understanding this fast-paced disorder and perhaps, one day, how to prevent it or slow its rate of progression. With every diagnosis of ALS that I make or confirm, and with every clinic visit, I try to put myself in the positions of the patient and caregiver. While this effort can only provide approximations of what the patient and caregiver experience, I hope it helps me see their issues and answer their questions in a realistic way. This book reflects what I would want to know and how I would want to be treated if I had ALS.

To further meet the needs of the patient, caregiver, and their family, I asked my coauthor, who is also my wife, to help me tell this story. We met when I treated her mother for ALS. Because she has worn the shoes of the caregiver, she brings a unique perspective on patient care and the patient viewpoint. That perspective has added a new dimension to my view of clinical experiences. We hope our unique combined voice will provide helpful guidance.

Mark B. Bromberg, MD, PhD

ACKNOWLEDGMENTS

I would like to express my thanks first to the patients whose questions I have endeavored to answer in this book. In particular I want to thank Creighton Rider, who has ALS, and his wife, Lisa, who provides his care, for reviewing the manuscript and providing valuable suggestions. I also want to acknowledge and thank my multidisciplinary colleagues who have guided the answers to many of the questions, including nurses (Dallas Forshew, Barbara Miano, Bernadette Talon, Mary Jensen, Cassie Kuhn, Abby Smart), a dietitian (Kari Lane), speech-language pathologists (Michelle Taggart, Kiera Berggren, Pamela Mathy), physical therapists (Nancy Ivy, Heather Hayes), occupational therapists (Kasey Mitchell, Jenny Ng), respiratory therapists (Natalie Bee, Aubrey Perman Isaacs), a genetic counselor (Karin Dent), social workers (Sandra Iaderosa, Kathy Day, Eva Tukuafu), clinic pharmacologists (Orly Vardeny, Kristen Jefferies, Patricia Jerant, Sarah Dehoney), a pulmonologist (Estelle Harris), a gastroenterologist (John Fang), and wheelchair seating specialists (Ron Whiting, Travis Carlson, Scott Ingraham). I am grateful to Craig Panner, editor at Oxford University Press, for asking us to write the book and helping with the editorial process.

Mark B. Bromberg, MD, PhD, FAAN

My contributions to this book reflect my personal rather than professional expertise, experiences, and views. I was very close to my parents throughout the course of my mother's illness, and I appreciate the opportunity to coauthor and add the caregiver perspective to this book. I have tried to supplement the medical information with the patient and caregiver points of view. I found that my approach to dealing with ALS was most often more practical than the physician's approach. Although mindful of the medical situation, my focus was usually on the emotional or day-to-day difficulties rather than strictly medical concerns. I believe the former aspects are as important to both patient and family as the medical consensus, in different ways. I also recognize that each patient and family situation is different, and that the practical impact on end-of-life treatments and financial issues will vary dramatically for each person. I thank my law partner, Jennifer Decker, for her input into the estate planning information we have provided.

I would also like to thank my parents. It is sometimes difficult to allow others to step in and help when a medical situation arises, but my parents not only welcomed the help but allowed me to share their fears, challenges, and frustrations during the course of my mother's illness. I hope that sharing the insights I gathered during that time will help patients, caregivers, and family members who are now dealing with ALS.

Diane Banks Bromberg, JD

Chapter 1

Introduction

What Are the Basic Features of ALS?

Amyotrophic lateral sclerosis (ALS) is a neurodegenerative disorder that mainly affects two types of **neurons** (nerve cells) that help control muscle movements and muscle strength: **upper motor neurons** and **lower motor neurons.** The terms "upper" and "lower" refer to nerve connections, with one group of nerves above connecting to another group of nerves below, and not to upper and lower limbs (Figure 1–1). When these nerve cells begin to degenerate and die, it is called **neurodegeneration.** The resulting weakness makes body and limb movements increasingly difficult. In some patients with ALS, degeneration of another set of nerve cells, which affect behavior and thinking, also occurs, resulting in **dementia.** These nerve cells are located in the front of the brain (**frontal lobes**) and the sides of the brain (**temporal lobes**), and the condition is called **frontotemporal lobe dementia (FTLD)** or **frontotemporal dementia (FTD)** (Figure 1–1).

ALS is a disease of adults, with onset most commonly in the sixth decade of life and rarely before the third and fourth decades. Men are affected slightly more commonly than women (Figure 1–2), and ALS affects individuals of all ethnic groups. The diagnosis is made or confirmed by a **neurologist,** who is a doctor trained in diagnosing and managing disorders of the nervous system. Optimal care is provided in **multidisciplinary ALS clinics.**

The cause of degeneration and death of upper motor neurons and lower motor neurons in ALS and FTLD is not known. No environmental factors, medical conditions, or life habits have been

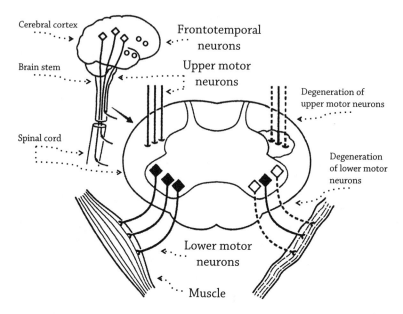

FIGURE 1-1 Neurons that degenerate and die in ALS. Upper left figure shows a side view of the brain as seen from the right, and lower figure shows a cross section of the spinal cord as viewed from above. Upper motor neurons are located in the cerebral cortex. They send their axons—the fibers that transmit their signals—to the brainstem and down the lateral sides of the spinal cord (lower figure, left side). Lower motor neurons are located in the spinal cord (and also in the brainstem) and send their axons to muscles (lower figure, left side). Death of upper motor neurons causes degeneration of axons in the lateral spinal tract (dashed lines, lower figure, right side). Death of lower motor neurons causes degeneration of axons to muscles and shrinkage of muscle (dashed lines, lower figure, right side). Neurons in the frontal and temporal lobes of the cerebral cortex (upper left figure) also degenerate in 50 percent of ALS patients.

identified as causes. In a small percentage of ALS patients, however, there is a **hereditary** factor, and for these individuals there is the possibility that ALS can be passed on to their children (see Chapter 4).

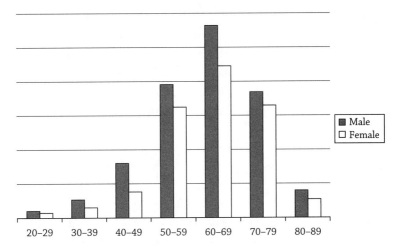

FIGURE 1–2 Age of symptom onset in ALS patients. Height of bars indicates relative frequency. Note that the disease has its peak onset in the sixth to seventh decades of life and affects more males than females.

Sadly, there is currently no medication that can stop or objectively slow the rate of nerve cell degeneration in ALS. Muscle weakness progresses, and patients most typically die as a result of difficulty breathing. Fifty percent of patients will die within 2 to 4 years after onset of their symptoms. Because deterioration is gradual, patients have time to make choices, and despite the challenges, most patients with ALS report a good quality of life.

During the course of ALS, muscle weakness causes symptoms or problems such as difficulty swallowing saliva and food, difficulty managing activities of daily living due to weakness of the hands and arms, difficulty with walking due to leg stiffness and weakness, and, in about 50 percent of patients, changes in behavior and mood due to FTLD. ALS does not affect sight, hearing, or other organs in the body, such as the heart, liver, or kidneys. It is not a painful disease, although discomfort may arise from not being able to move and change positions. Thankfully, a number of aids are available that can make people more comfortable and help them to live longer.

Many medical centers have special multidisciplinary ALS clinics where a range of **healthcare providers**, such as **speech-language pathologists, occupational therapists, physical therapists, respiratory therapists**, and **dietitians**, can offer a full range of support and care. Since caregiver burden increases as ALS progresses, a multidisciplinary clinic will also have a **nurse** and **social worker** to assist caregivers.

Not only do these clinics provide medical information, but they also fill a niche for both patients and caregivers, who look forward to appointments as times to get updates on the patient's condition and ask questions. It is common to forget to ask questions during these appointments, so many patients and caregivers find it helpful to keep a written list of questions that arise between clinic visits and review them during the visit. It is useful for the caregiver and family members to accompany the patient to each visit to ensure that the full range of issues is addressed, and it is also appropriate to address caregiver questions and needs during clinic visits. Many communities have **support groups** where patients and caregivers can exchange ideas and concerns and obtain useful information.

How It Starts: Patient Stories

The onset of ALS is different for each patient. Weakness starts focally (affecting movement at one site—for example, speech or movement of a hand or leg), and over time spreads to affect other regions of the body. Despite differences in the initial site of appearance, neurologists recognize a pattern of loss of both upper and lower motor neurons over time. Although there is no specific diagnostic test for ALS, the clinical features are unique, and the diagnosis can be made with confidence.

Just as every patient's onset of weakness differs, so too does recognition of the problem. These initial differences are illustrated by the following patient and caregiver stories. The first three pairs of patients and caregivers are hypothetical but are based on real experiences and designed to cover the broad spectrum of ALS presentations. The fourth patient story is that of the coauthor's mother. These same patients and caregivers will appear throughout the book as they manage the challenges of ALS.

The first patient had initial difficulty with speech.

Hello, I am Betty and just turned 65. I first noted difficulty singing in church. There was a cold going around, and I thought I had the "bug" even though I did not have sniffles or a cough. I practiced in the shower, but my voice would crack. A few months later, friends asked if I had a head cold, as my voice had changed. At meals I began drinking a second glass of water to help clear my swallow before the next bite. I was horribly embarrassed when, during a phone conversation with my best friend, she asked if I'd been drinking alcohol, because my speech was slurred.

Betty's problems with singing, speaking, and swallowing were related, as all require a series of complex and interactive muscle movements.

Henry here—Betty's other half. She was the songbird of our church's choir, always hitting the high notes. That began to change, and she became so embarrassed she dropped out of the choir. She was depressed about the changes and was no longer interested in going to church. I had to practically drag her there. She tended to cry easily, and I could not console her. In thinking back after the diagnosis, I recognized there had been a change in her personality over the past year, in that she became quiet, spoke with few words, and was easily irritated.

(Continued)

(*Continued*)

Our son called to ask what was wrong because he couldn't understand the voice messages she left for him. Our daughter visited from out of town and was shocked at the change in her mother over the 6-month interval since she'd last seen her. When our daughter told me she was frightened, I realized I was too. We went to five different kinds of doctors before Betty was finally diagnosed with ALS by a neurologist. During this time Betty became more and more withdrawn, quiet, and easily irritated. The neurologist explained that such changes can be part of ALS.

Our next patient began with difficulty using his hands for fine motor activities.

My name is John and I am 58. I first had a problem buttoning my collar when dressing for work. I thought it was a particularly tight shirt, but I had the same problem almost every day, even though I wore a different shirt each time. Then it became hard to turn the key to start the car. It was late winter, and I thought my cold hand was the problem. The muscles in my hand also cramped up, and I had to use the other hand to stretch them out. That had never happened to me before. One night I was trying to untwist a jar cap and could not do it. My wife jokingly asked to try it, and she had no difficulty. We then looked at my hands more closely, and some muscles were shrunken.

A family member may be first to tie changes in function to the possibility of illness.

I am John's wife, Carol. John is a can-do type of guy and has never asked for help with much of anything. I was more than a little surprised when he started needing help with buttons. I first thought maybe he had gained a little weight, so I bought him shirts with larger collars. But that didn't help. I really became concerned when he could not open the jar cap. We talked about his hand muscles shrinking and decided he should see a doctor.

The third patient had difficulty walking.

I am Stephen, and I began falling. I retired three years ago, when I was 65, so that I could spend more time outside. I like to work in the yard, which is large and sloping, and take pride in landscaping. I had no difficulty behind the lawn mower but noticed I couldn't easily walk up and down the most sloping parts without holding onto the mower for balance. My wife commented that I was walking slower, and friends asked if my right knee was OK because I seemed to favor it. One time I fell in the yard and could not get up without crawling to a tree and using it for support. That night I talked to my wife, and she admitted she had also noted changes over the past few months. She also mentioned that when she lies close to me in bed, she feels small jerks in my muscles. I have noted them too.

Sometimes the person's partner begins to investigate what the problem may be and suspects the diagnosis even before a doctor is seen.

Stephen and I have a big yard that is our pet project. Oh, I am his wife, Rachel. We love working in the yard almost daily during the season, and he knows the yard like the back of his hand. When he started tripping and falling when doing yard work we could not understand why. At first it was once in a while, and then more often. He walked more stiffly and slowly and laughed it off as old age, but we obviously did not think age was the cause when he fell and could not get up. He was only 68. When I noted muscle twitches at night I did a search on the computer to see if I could figure it out. His twitching and falling fit with ALS: what a shock! I was not surprised when the third doctor we saw diagnosed ALS. I was even proud that I figured it out before we went to that doctor, but it was a bittersweet success.

Our fourth and final patient's problems were first overlooked, until a series of falls made them hard to ignore.

I am Diane. When my mother, Lois, was 78 years old she became very difficult to understand on the telephone. Since she lived in a rural area and I lived in the city, we talked on the phone and left voice messages frequently. Even my boys started to remark that you couldn't understand her voice messages. I don't know why we didn't look into her problems further at this point, but when she tripped and fell on vacation and again at church, we became concerned enough to see a doctor. We started with an internist. It was a surprise to me when the doctor's examination focused mostly on Mom's walking and balance. I guess I expected some simple solution or procedure instead of the challenging

(Continued)

> *(Continued)*
> disease we were dealing with. That first doctor sent us to
> a neurologist, who diagnosed ALS on the first visit and
> sent us to a second neurologist who specializes in ALS for
> confirmation.

From these four patient histories of early ALS symptoms one can get a feeling for how ALS may first appear. One site of neuro-degeneration is in the **bulbar region** of the brain, which resides in the **brainstem**, just below the **cerebral cortex** (also called the cerebral hemispheres). It gets its name because to early neurologists it looked like a tulip bulb. Upper motor neurons to and lower motor neurons from this region control the tongue and lips for speech and the muscles for swallowing. Accordingly, degeneration here causes about one-third of patients to first have speech and swallowing difficulties. Betty, our first patient above, presented with bulbar-onset ALS.

Another common site is the **cervical spine region**. In this region upper motor neuron fibers run downwards, and lower motor neurons leave from here to control muscles of the hand and arm. Another one-third of ALS patients present with upper limb onset, as did John, our second patient.

Difficulties can start with leg stiffness and weakness for another one-third of patients, like Stephen, our third patient. For him, stiffness of walking was due to fewer upper motor neurons reaching the **lumbosacral spine region**, and leg muscle weakness was due to fewer lower motor neurons in this region. Lois's weakness started with bulbar symptoms, similar to Betty, and shortly thereafter progressed to her lumbosacral spine region.

Once the diagnosis is made, the symptoms and patient difficulties fall into place. In a large percentage of patients, ALS also affects behavior, in ways that may be subtle. Betty became withdrawn and lost interest in activities, such as going to church, that were previously important for her. This likely was due to loss of neurons in the frontal and temporal regions of the brain (FTLD).

As we have seen, the minor problems in the beginning are frequently ignored, and the patient often passes them off as insignificant or finds an excuse to explain them. But as time goes on and the problems become greater, there is a point when they can no longer be ignored. The time from first symptoms to a diagnosis of ALS averages 9 to 12 months, depending on the speed of progression and the experience of the doctors who are consulted. If the progression is rapid, the patient will typically see a doctor sooner than if progression is slow. The first doctor may not recognize early signs of ALS and may send the patient to another doctor. A doctor may think that the presenting problem is due to a pinched nerve and recommend that the patient see a surgeon. Given the severity of ALS, a neurologist may recommend a second opinion, and it is actually not uncommon for a patient to see four to six doctors before the diagnosis is confirmed.

How to Use This Book

This book is divided into three sections. In **Chapters 2 to 6** we answer basic questions and concerns of patients and family members: What is ALS, and what are the subtypes? How is it diagnosed? What do we know about causes? Who gets ALS, and why me? Will I pass it on to my children? In **Chapters 7 to 13** we discuss in greater detail what happens once ALS is diagnosed and how to manage symptoms. In **Chapters 14 to 16** we discuss the role of the caregiver, end-of-life issues, and planning ahead. **Chapter 17** considers research. The final chapter, **Chapter 18,** is a reflection on the whole of ALS. Throughout, we will follow Betty, John, Stephen, and Lois; their partners; and their families as they live with ALS.

ALS is a most challenging disease; though it affects patients in similar ways overall, each patient is nonetheless different and their families will react differently. Patients, caregivers, and family members will likely have similar questions, but each may also have unique questions. This book tries to cover a wide spectrum of patient and caregiver experiences and their questions. The reader may want to quickly look over the book for an overview of ALS and then go back to earlier parts as new issues and questions arise. Readers should use the book in tandem with the information they receive from the patient's own medical professionals. Multidisciplinary ALS clinics have been established to optimize care, and patients are encouraged to seek out such a clinic.

Finally, it is important to understand that no patient with ALS has all the symptoms described in this book, and no two patients follow the same course.

A special vocabulary of terms and abbreviations is associated with ALS. As you may have noticed, important terms are shown in bold; these are defined in the **Glossary** at the end of the book.

Chapter 2

ALS Origins

Why the Name ALS?

ALS stands for "amyotrophic lateral sclerosis." The words come from the French *sclérose latérale amyotrophique*. "**Amyotrophic**" indicates the presence of **atrophy**, or shrinkage, of muscles due to loss of lower motor neurons, which are the nerves that go from the brainstem and **spinal cord** to muscles; "lateral" refers to the sides of the spinal cord; and "**sclerosis**" refers to hardening from scar tissue, which occurs when there is a loss of upper motor neurons that send their fibers along the lateral sides of the spinal cord (see Figure 1–1). The features of ALS were first recognized and written about in the mid-1800s. The French neurologist Jean-Martin Charcot observed under the microscope that there was loss of upper and lower motor neurons and gave the disease its descriptive name.

Is ALS Different from Motor Neuron Disease?

Motor neuron disease (MND) is the term used to cover all forms of diseases of the motor neurons. Such diseases include ALS as well as **primary lateral sclerosis (PLS), progressive muscular atrophy (PMA), and progressive bulbar palsy (PBP)**. They are grouped together because they are characterized by loss of upper and lower motor neurons, although to different degrees: PLS and PBP involve only loss of upper motor neurons, PMA involves only loss of lower motor neurons, but ALS involves loss of both upper and lower motor

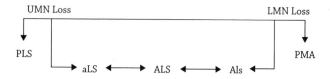

FIGURE 2-1 Spectrum of upper motor neuron (UMN) and lower motor neuron (LMN) loss among patients with ALS. Primary lateral sclerosis (PLS) denotes patients with only UMN loss. Progressive muscular atrophy (PMA) denotes patients with only LMN loss. aLS, ALS, and Als denote patients with different relative amounts of upper and lower motor neuron loss.

neurons to varying degrees (Figure 2–1). Patients may start with PLS or PBP (loss of upper motor neurons) or PMA (loss of lower motor neurons), but almost all progress over months to ALS (loss of both upper and lower motor neurons). The term MND is used interchangeably with ALS in the United Kingdom.

Many patients report that they had never heard the term ALS or did not know much about it before their diagnosis.

Is ALS a New or Old Disease?

ALS is not a new disease, as it was described in the 1800s and thus existed before that time. We also know this because rare hereditary forms of ALS, called **familial ALS (fALS)**, exist where gene mutations are passed down family lines. For some genes, calculations have been made to answer the question of how old or how far back in time the hereditary forms go. Some gene mutations in ALS represent events with a founder, or "Adam-Eve," effect. That is, a single person had a spontaneous gene mutation and passed it on to his or her offspring, who in turn passed it on, and so forth, down generations. Calculations made on the number of generations involved show that for some ALS gene mutations, the first person affected likely goes back as far as 6,000 or more years. Although similar calculations cannot be made for **sporadic ALS** (ALS in individuals with no affected family members), it is also likely to have existed for a very long time.

How Common Is ALS?

ALS is considered to be a rare disease. The US Centers for Disease Control and Prevention (CDC) defines a disease as rare when fewer than 200,000 persons are affected in the United States during one year; the estimated prevalence of ALS in the United States is approximately 35,000 affected people per year. The estimated incidence is about 2/100,000: this means that every year two people in 100,000 will develop ALS. Another way to look at these data is that the lifetime risk of developing ALS is about 1 in 350 for men and 1 in 450 for women. In the United States, a person is diagnosed with ALS every 90 minutes. For fALS, the risk will be higher (see Chapter 4).

Who Was Lou Gehrig?

In the United States, ALS is commonly known as Lou Gehrig's disease. Lou Gehrig was a baseball player for the New York Yankees who was also known as the "iron horse" because of his all-around skills and his record of playing in 2,130 consecutive games. He first noticed his fatigue midway through the 1938 season, at the age of 35. His performance was off at the start of 1939, and he received the diagnosis of ALS that spring. He retired from baseball that year and on July 4, 1939, gave his well-known farewell speech in Yankee Stadium (Figure 2–2), which included his statement "Fans, for the past two weeks you have been reading about the bad break I got. Yet today I consider myself the luckiest man on the face of this earth." He died in 1941.

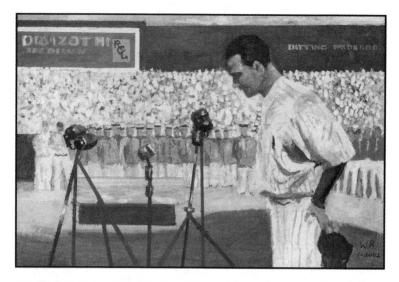

FIGURE 2–2 Lou Gehrig's farewell speech at Yankee Stadium on July 4, 1939, as shown in a watercolor titled *Pride of the Yankees* by William Ross, who has ALS. Ross painted the picture with a brush held in his mouth because of limb weakness. From the Muscular Dystrophy Association art collection, with permission.

Who Else Had ALS?

ALS has affected people in all walks of life, in all parts of the world, and of all ethnic groups. Internationally known people who had ALS are listed in Table 2–1. Professor Stephen Hawking is not included on the list, as he is still alive. A common question is, why has he lived so long with ALS? Professor Hawking's medical record is private, but information about his condition can be obtained from the Internet to answer questions surrounding the course of his illness. He is 74 years old as of this writing. He developed difficulty walking around age 20 and he states that he received a diagnosis of ALS at age 21. His speech and limb movements have deteriorated, requiring him to rely upon computer aids for communication and 24-hour

TABLE 2–1 Internationally Known People Who Had ALS

Lou Gehrig: Baseball player

Jim "Catfish" Hunter: Baseball player

Bruce Edwards: Professional golf caddy

Henry Wallace: 33rd Vice President of the United States

Maxwell Taylor: US Army general

Jacob Javits: US senator (New York)

Mao Zedong: Leader, People's Republic of China

Jon Stone: Writer, producer of *Sesame Street*

Dmitri Shostakovich: Composer

Huddie Ledbetter (Lead Belly): Musician

Charles Mingus: Jazz pianist

David Niven: Actor

Lane Smith: Actor

Dennis Day: TV personality

Morrie Schwartz: Educator (subject of the book *Tuesdays with Morrie*)

care for the past 30 years. While he has lived for over 50 years since the diagnosis, he had respiratory failure in 1985 and has been dependent upon a ventilator for the past 30 years. The natural course of his ALS would have been approximately 20 years without artificial ventilation.

Chapter 3

The Diagnosis of ALS

ALS is a unique disease, and no single laboratory test results in a clear "yes/no" diagnosis. Instead the diagnosis of ALS is a *clinical diagnosis* based on the history of how problems started and the pattern of progression, the neurologic examination, and a few informative laboratory tests. This chapter will help the patient and family to understand the process of making a clinical diagnosis. There are three clinical features specific to ALS:

- Evidence for upper motor neuron degeneration
- Evidence for lower motor neuron degeneration
- Evidence for progression, within a region and to other regions of the body

What Does the Neurologist Look for?

The neurologist takes a history, performs a neurologic examination, and then may order laboratory tests. The most important aspect is the patient's history of symptoms. *Symptoms* are the problems that a patient has experienced or is experiencing and that cause the patient to visit the doctor. During the taking of the history, the neurologist listens for evidence of the three features listed above. During the neurologic examination the neurologist looks for signs that confirm loss of upper and lower motor neurons. *Signs* are abnormalities observed from testing muscle function and strength, watching the patient walk, and testing tendon reflexes. A tendon reflex is the jerk of a muscle when the neurologist taps the attached tendon with a reflex hammer. Laboratory tests are used to verify lower motor neuron loss, but there are no laboratory tests to verify upper motor neuron loss. Other tests may be ordered and are discussed below.

What Are the Symptoms and Signs of ALS?

Symptoms and signs of ALS depend at any given time on the degree of upper and lower motor loss and the regions of the body that are affected. Table 3–1 lists difficulties patients experience based on whether loss of upper or lower motor neurons is responsible, but it

TABLE 3-1 Symptoms Patients Describe and Signs Neurologists Find during the Diagnostic Examination That Support Upper and Lower Motor Neuron Loss

Upper Motor Neuron Loss		*Lower Motor Neuron Loss*	
Symptoms	*Signs*	*Symptoms*	*Signs*
Bulbar Region		*Bulbar Region*	
• Slurred speech	• Spastic speech	• Muscle shrinkage	• Muscle atrophy
• Difficulty swallowing	• Choking while drinking	• Weakness	• Muscle weakness upon testing
Arms and Legs		*Arms and Legs*	
• Slow movements	• Slow development of strength	• Muscle twitches	• Fasciculations
• Unsteady walking	• Spastic gait	• Muscle cramps	• Cramps during muscle testing
	• Jumpy tendon reflexes		• Characteristic findings on EMG study

is important to appreciate that symptoms can be due to a combination of upper and lower motor neuron loss.

Bulbar Difficulties

Patients describe slurring of words or the need to work harder to form words. This problem occurs with **spastic** speech due to upper motor neuron loss. Patients also describe early difficulty with swallowing, such as the need for several swallows to clear food and greater difficulties swallowing liquids, which is also due to upper motor neuron loss. It may also be difficult to use the tongue effectively to clear food between the cheek and teeth due to lower motor neuron loss.

During the examination, the neurologist listens for slurred speech. When speech is slurred, inspection of the tongue is informative because a weak tongue with tongue atrophy (shrinkage of muscle) supports slurring that is due to lower motor neuron loss, while an absence of tongue atrophy supports slurring due to upper motor neuron loss. There may be components of both upper and lower motor neuron loss when speech is slurred.

Upper Extremity Difficulties

The patient may also report weakness in hand and arm muscles, which is more commonly due to lower motor neuron loss. Brief twitches of muscles, called **fasciculations**, may be noted by the patient or the patient's partner, and patients may also describe an increase in muscle cramps or cramps in unusual muscles; all of these symptoms support lower motor neuron loss. Additionally, the patient may describe slow movements of the arms, and fingers may move with less dexterity, both of which are symptoms supporting upper motor neuron loss.

The neurologist looks for weakness and for signs of muscle atrophy. Certain muscles in the hand are more commonly involved than others, and the patient may not be aware of such involvement. Lower motor nerves that go to muscles in the hand on the thumb side are affected before those on the little-finger side, and this is referred to as the **split hand syndrome**. This pattern of atrophy and weakness is unique to ALS and is one sign the neurologist focuses on. Observation for fasciculations, which the patient may not be aware of, is important, as they represent lower motor neuron loss. Clinical signs of upper motor neuron loss affecting the upper extremities are stiffness of the arm to bending at the elbow (spasticity) and hyperactive tendon reflexes.

Lower Extremity Difficulties

Difficulty walking is the lower extremity symptom that often brings the patient to the doctor. Most commonly the patient describes poor balance and "hard falls" due to not being able to regain balance after tripping. This suggests leg stiffness (spasticity) from upper motor neuron loss. A **footdrop** (weakness at the ankle causing the foot to drag) often results in tripping and suggests lower motor neuron loss. Another symptom of lower motor neuron loss is difficulty rising from a chair due to thigh muscle weakness and giving out of the leg at the knee when walking. Fasciculations and cramps may also occur in the legs.

Clinical signs of lower motor neuron loss that the neurologist looks for in the lower extremities are muscle atrophy and weakness. Upper motor neuron signs are stiff or spastic gait and hyperactive tendon reflexes.

Progression of Symptoms

The pattern of progression of weakness is important, and the neurologist will ask about progression from when the patient first noted difficulties to the time of the clinic visit. ALS starts focally, meaning that it begins with weakness or difficulties with movement in one part or area of the body. Weakness and difficulties increase in severity within the first region and then move to other parts of the body. In most cases, the weakness in the arms or legs starts asymmetrically (on one side) and then goes to the other side. For instance, initial difficulty using the right hand while everything remains normal with the left will be followed, after the passage of time, with similar weakness in the left hand. A similar pattern of progression occurs in leg muscles. However, weakness can also move from an arm to a leg, or vice versa, before involving a limb on the other side. If difficulties first occur with speech, then arms or legs are affected next. Few if any other diseases progress along this pattern.

Two features uniquely associated with ALS, pseudobulbar affect and elements of FTLD, also help secure the diagnosis of ALS when present. Both conditions are discussed in greater detail in Chapter 6.

To return to three of our patients and their stories from Chapter 1, Betty began with upper motor neuron loss affecting her singing, and her difficulties progressed to her conversational speech and then to her swallowing. Later she developed weakness of her hand muscles due to lower motor neuron loss before the diagnosis of ALS was made. Her withdrawal from socializing demonstrated that she also had features of FTLD. Stephen began with stiffness of walking (spasticity) with frequent falling due to upper motor neuron loss. He soon thereafter developed atrophy and weakness of leg muscles and hand muscles due to loss of lower motor neurons. John first noted atrophy and weakness of hand and arm muscles from lower motor neuron loss and upon examination also had evidence for upper motor neuron loss.

What Are the Most Important Tests?

Although no single laboratory test can confirm the diagnosis of ALS, the most important test to aid in the diagnosis is the **electrodiagnostic test**, which consists of **nerve conduction test** and the needle **electromyography (EMG) test**. These studies are performed in an EMG laboratory in a neurologist's office or in a laboratory at a medical center. Nerve conduction tests record responses from sensory and motor nerves and are performed by taping electrodes over nerves or muscles (similar to the electrodes taped to the chest to record heart rhythms during electrocardiogram [ECG or EKG] recordings). The nerves are activated by brief electrical shocks delivered to the skin that overlies the nerves. Nerve conduction tests can ensure that only motor nerves (and not sensory nerves) are involved and can rule out other disorders that might look like ALS.

The needle EMG study is the most sensitive test for determining which muscles are affected by lower motor neuron loss. The EMG study is performed by a neurologist, who inserts a small needle electrode into various muscles, which records the electrical activity generated in the muscles when the patient gently activates (contracts) the muscles. The signals are analyzed to look for changes due to loss of lower motor neurons. The EMG can show early loss of nerves to a muscle before it becomes clinically atrophic and weak. A muscle becomes weak only after more than 50 percent of the lower motor nerves going to the muscle have degenerated and died. As the first half of the nerves degenerate, the remaining ones can compensate; it is only when there are too few remaining nerves to compensate that the muscle becomes weak. However, the EMG study can detect the compensation process and hence can show progression away from the initial site of weakness and to other sites. Showing that lower motor neuron loss is occurring in a diffusely distributed pattern is a unique feature of ALS.

What Are the El Escorial Criteria?

Neurologists making the diagnosis of ALS may mention the **El Escorial criteria**. These criteria represent an effort by the World Federation of Neurology to aid in formalizing the diagnosis of ALS.

(El Escorial is the city in Spain where the conference was held.) The diagnostic levels of "definite," "probable," and "possible" ALS indicate the distribution of upper and lower motor neuron signs at that time. These labels are used to ensure that consistent groups of patients are entered in drug trials for ALS. The El Escorial criteria are also used in the clinic as guidelines to confirm the diagnosis. The levels are generally determined at the time of diagnosis, and as weakness progresses patients can move from one category to another. It is important to understand that the categories do not indicate differing degrees of doubt about the diagnosis.

What Are "Rule Out" Tests?

Some doctors order a large number of laboratory tests to "rule out" any other diagnosis, and when all those test results are normal, conclude that the patient has ALS. Essentially no diseases truly mimic ALS if a careful medical and neurologic history is taken and a careful neurologic examination is performed. While it may seem reassuring that all tests have been performed, in reality it raises false hope that another diagnosis will be reached. In addition, false-positive test results can occur (results with abnormal values that turn out not to be related to a diagnosis different from ALS), again giving false hope. Finally, testing can be uncomfortable (sometimes even painful) and is costly.

Below are tests some neurologists may order, but research does not support an alternative diagnosis to ALS based solely on abnormal values from these tests:

- Complete blood count (CBC)
- Electrolytes (sodium, potassium, chloride)
- Creatine kinase (CK or CPK)
- Antibodies associated with autoimmune diseases (Antinuclear antigens [ANA], rheumatoid factor [RF])

- Elevated serum protein (monoclonal protein)
- Antibodies associated with peripheral neuropathies (anti-GM1 gangliosides)
- Heavy metals (lead, mercury, arsenic, thallium) in blood or urine
- Lumbar puncture with analysis of spinal fluid
- Muscle biopsy
- Magnetic resonance imaging (MRI) scans of the brain, cervical spine, thoracic spine, lumbosacral spine

In the end, it is up to the neurologist making the diagnosis to be confident that the diagnosis is correct.

Why Does Making the Diagnosis Take So Much Time?

The time it takes to make the diagnosis of ALS varies among patients. One factor is the time from symptom onset to the time a patient seeks medical evaluation. Some patients seek medical attention early on while others wait to see if the problem might get better on its own. Waiting may be more common if the progression of weakness is slow; fewer people wait if the progression is more rapid. Another factor influencing when the diagnosis is made is whether the first doctor the patient saw thought of ALS or referred the patient to specialists looking for another cause. It is not uncommon for a primary care doctor to refer a patient with speech and swallowing difficulties to a doctor who specializes in ear, nose, and throat disorders (an otolaryngologist) or a patient with hand or leg function difficulties to an orthopedic surgeon who looks for issues in the spine. Sometimes orthopedists recommend and perform surgery in the hopes of fixing the difficulty. Sometimes the patient consults three or four doctors before seeing a neurologist. Finally, some neurologists suggest or patients request a second opinion by another neurologist. Overall, it takes an average of 9 to 12 months, measured from the onset of the first symptoms, and three to six doctors to make a diagnosis of ALS.

It is estimated that primary care physicians may see one or two ALS patients in their careers, and thus they are not always familiar with the various early symptoms. Efforts are being made to educate primary care physicians to be alert to "red flags" in a patient's history and examination in order to shorten the time to diagnosis. The El Escorial criteria are also an effort to refine criteria to enable patients to be diagnosed more quickly. These efforts, however, do not reduce the time it takes for a patient to seek medical attention.

Do I Really Have ALS? What Diseases Mimic ALS?

Everyone who seeks medical attention for difficulties suggestive of ALS hopes that he or she does not have ALS but rather a disease that mimics ALS but is treatable. While ALS is a unique disease, other diseases are frequently considered during the diagnostic process.

Multifocal Motor Neuropathy with Conduction Block

Multifocal motor neuropathy with conduction block (MMN) is a very rare form of neuropathy that affects motor nerves and can be treated, leading to improvement in strength. It is associated with the special feature of focal **conduction block** of nerve impulses. When nerve impulses are blocked, the muscle does not receive the intended message and appears to be weak. Features of MMN that may make doctors think of that diagnosis and not ALS include the fact that MMN affects single nerves, one at a time, and thus has an asymmetric pattern. In addition, muscles may be atrophic, and patients may notice fasciculations. Conduction block is demonstrated during nerve conduction studies but is frequently overinterpreted when in fact there is no block.

MMN has very different clinical features from ALS. It does not include degeneration of upper motor neurons, and tendon reflexes are normal and not pathologic. The muscles affected tend to be different from those affected in ALS. MMN has a stepwise progression, and progression is slower (taking many years) than in ALS. Further, there is no pseudobulbar affect or FTLD. A large number of patients with ALS have been treated for possible MMN, but with no improvement in strength.

Inclusion Body Myositis

Inclusion body myositis (IBM) is a primary muscle disease. Clinical similarities with ALS include weakness starting when the person is more than 50 years old, asymmetric muscle atrophy and weakness, and occasional muscle cramps and fasciculations. However, the distribution of muscle weakness and atrophy is different from that in ALS: IBM uniquely affects muscles in the forearm responsible for grip and thigh muscles responsible for rising from a chair and keeping from falling while walking. Progression is very slow, over many years. Further, reflexes are normal, and there is no pseudobulbar affect or FTLD.

Kennedy Disease

Kennedy disease, also known as spinal bulbar muscular atrophy, is a very rare genetic form of motor neuron disease that is X-linked, thus affecting men only (see Chapter 4 for information on genetic transmission). There is loss of lower motor neurons but not upper motor neurons, and also loss of sensory neurons. Thus patients present with difficulty speaking and swallowing, with weakness in a symmetric distribution, and numbness and tingling in their arms and legs. Tendon reflexes are absent. Interestingly, many men with spinal bulbar muscular atrophy have enlarged breast tissue. It is a very slowly progressive form of motor neuron disease, and an occasional male patient will be told that he has ALS but, after living longer than predicted, will be discovered to actually have Kennedy disease. A gene test is available to make a definitive diagnosis of Kennedy disease.

Cervical Spondylitic Myelopathy

Cervical spondylitic myelopathy is the name given to changes in the neck (cervical spine) due to bony enlargement and disk degeneration. It is thought that the bony changes can cause a narrowing of the spinal canal with pressure on the spinal cord (**myelopathy**), with results that mimic upper motor neuron signs of ALS, and pressure on motor roots as they leave the spine, with results that mimic lower motor neuron signs of ALS.

Patterns of involvement in cervical spondylitic myelopathy are different from those in ALS. First, in cervical spondylitic myelopathy the upper motor neuron signs come from the spinal cord and exclude any of the bulbar (speech and swallowing) difficulties, pseudobulbar affect, or FTLD frequently observed in ALS. Second, the pattern of arm and hand weakness is different from that in ALS. Usually, marked pain that shoots from the neck down the arm is present and rarely affects both arms. Third, cervical spine difficulties cannot explain any weakness or EMG changes noted in the legs (which occur in ALS). Older patients may have both cervical spondylitic myelopathy and ALS; many such patients have undergone cervical spine surgery in the hopes that they would become stronger, but surgery almost never results in any improvement or slowing of the progression of ALS.

Lumbosacral Spondylitic Radiculopathy

Similar pathology from bony changes and disk degeneration can occur in the lumbosacral spine region as in the neck, causing pressure on nerves going to the legs. However, because the spinal cord ends farther up in the back, no upper motor neuron signs due to lower spine bony pathology are present in lumbosacral spondylitic radiculopathy. Similar to what occurs with neck pathology, marked pains that shoot down the leg (sciatica) are usually present. Further, lumbosacral spine pathology cannot explain weakness or EMG changes in the arms (which occur in ALS). As with cervical spondylitic conditions, older patients may have both conditions, but low back spine surgery has not resulted in improvement of leg weakness due to ALS.

Lyme Disease

Lyme disease is caused by a bacterial infection transmitted by a bite from a tick, the insect that carries the bacterium. Infected ticks are found in limited regions of the country (the name "Lyme disease" comes from a town in Connecticut), and Lyme disease can cause a number of symptoms, including neurologic problems. However, a clinical picture of upper and lower motor neuron loss with progression is not one of them. Lyme disease can sometimes be diagnosed by blood tests, but the tests document exposure to the bacterium and not unsuspected current infection. When classic symptoms appear, treatment by antibiotics is appropriate and clears the body of the infection. There is the notion of "chronic Lyme disease," resulting in prolonged treatment periods, but if the disease is ALS rather than Lyme disease, such prolonged treatment will not result in patients getting better.

Carpal Tunnel Syndrome

Carpal tunnel syndrome is caused by pressure on the median nerve as it passes through the wrist. It most commonly causes numbness and tingling of fingers (from the thumb through part of the ring finger), but some patients may interpret weakness in fingers as numbness. Patients may have carpal tunnel release surgery with the hope of improvement, but it is not successful in ALS, because the affected nerves are in the spinal cord and not at the wrist.

Ulnar Neuropathy at the Elbow

The ulnar nerve crosses the elbow and activates several muscles in the hand (in particular, the muscle in the web between the thumb and second finger) that are commonly weak and atrophic early in ALS. Sometimes a surgical release procedure at the elbow reduces the pressure on the nerve that causes ulnar neuropathy, but such a procedure is not successful in ALS, because the nerves affected in ALS are in the spinal cord and not at the elbow.

Should I Get a Second Opinion?

Many patients see several physicians before receiving the diagnosis of ALS. Frequently, the last doctor seen before the neurologist who gives the diagnosis has a strong suspicion of the diagnosis, and the neurologist's confirmation can be viewed as another opinion. However, the most important issue is whether the patient and family are confident in the diagnosis. A neurologist is the most knowledgeable person to give the diagnosis. If a second opinion from another neurologist would make the patient and family more comfortable, it is suggested that the second neurologist be one who has extensive experience with ALS; such as neurologists in ALS clinics in major medical centers.

How Was the Diagnosis Given and Received?

No doctor wants to give the diagnosis of ALS, and no patient wants to receive it. There have been efforts among ALS neurologists to give the diagnosis of ALS in person, in a gentle manner, and with time to explain the disease and answer questions, and to provide written material for the patient and family to review. An experienced neurologist may not be the first person mentioning or giving the diagnosis, and thus the patient may not have been given the diagnosis with full consideration of how it might be received. Unfortunately, this can leave a lasting negative impression on the patient and family.

Occasionally patients or family members will be deeply upset about receiving a diagnosis of such a challenging disease and will be angry with the neurologist no matter how the diagnosis was presented. These feelings may be managed by a second opinion or with the passage of time. Sometimes the feelings interfere with working with the neurologist, and if so, discussing them within the family and with the ALS clinic social worker can help.

Chapter 4

Causes of ALS

What Causes ALS?

Simply stated, the cause of ALS is not known. It is possible that the clinical condition of ALS actually represents a number of different diseases that start from different causes but follow a pathway that converges. For example, we know that there are at least two forms of ALS: familial ALS (fALS), where the disease can be passed down in the family, and sporadic ALS (sALS), where there is no family history. Within fALS, different **genes** may be involved, and likely each gene causes different initial changes in motor neurons that lead to their degeneration and death. Furthermore, since ALS begins with symptoms at different regions (bulbar, arm, leg) and with different degrees of involvement of upper motor neurons and lower motor neurons (PLS and PMA), these variations could represent different forms of motor neuron disease (MND). In addition, different time courses of progression are observed among patients, from a very short time (first symptom to death in 1 year) to very long time courses (over 10 years), which could also be due to different mechanisms of nerve cell death.

It is important to note that despite differences among patients—fALS or sALS, site of onset, degree of upper and lower motor neuron involvement, and time course—all patients have a recognizable clinical pattern supporting the diagnosis of ALS. Thus it is likely that a number of causative factors (reviewed below) lead to a sequence of pathologic changes in neurons that ultimately leads to a "final common pathway" of degeneration and death of upper and lower motor neurons.

Why Do Neurons Die in ALS?

ALS is one of several neurodegenerative diseases. Other common neurodegenerative diseases include Alzheimer disease and Parkinson disease. All are characterized by sets of neurons, particular to each disease, that degenerate and die. We do not know why only specific neurons die for each disease or what goes wrong to start the process of neuron degeneration leading to neuron death. So why mention other neurodegenerative diseases? There are two primary reasons: one is to emphasize that the causes remain unknown for all neurodegenerative diseases, and the other is that because of similarities among neurodegenerative diseases, research on one of these diseases can help in understanding the others.

A number of theories as to why neurons die in ALS will be discussed in this chapter, but it is important to note that at this time in our understanding of ALS, all are just theories. Data exist to support each theory, and drugs have been tested in ALS based on the theories, but the drug trials have not been successful. This does not mean that the theories are incorrect. For example, a drug may not have reached the right place in the nervous system, or the right dose of the drug was not achieved. Furthermore, each theory is not exclusive of another theory, and the theories may each represent a step in a cascade of events leading to neuron death. Because patients often read about new discoveries and treatments based on these theories, it is useful to briefly present a number of them.

Glutamate Excitotoxicity

Nerve cells interact with other nerve cells when the first cell secretes a **neurotransmitter** that crosses a tiny gap (called the **synapse**) to excite or activate the next cell. **Glutamate** is the neurotransmitter that activates upper and lower motor neurons. One theory is that in ALS there is a relative excess of glutamate that could be toxic to upper and lower motor neurons. Support for this is that in a laboratory setting, very high levels of glutamate can cause nerve cells to die. This is called **excitotoxicity**. This relative excess would occur only at the synapse between nerve cells, and the level of glutamate cannot be measured in patients with ALS.

A question patients often ask in this context is whether the food spice monosodium glutamate could increase glutamate in the brain. The answer is no, because glutamate used as a neurotransmitter comes from sources within the body and not from the diet.

Oxidative Stress

Oxidative stress is a natural process occurring in all cells. There are mechanisms within cells to manage cellular stress. It is possible that excess oxidative stress occurs in ALS. Excess glutamate (glutamate excitotoxicity) could increase oxidative stress.

Mitochondrial Dysfunction

Energy is required for all biochemical activities in cells, and a major source of this energy is produced by **mitochondria**, tiny structures in every cell. If mitochondria are damaged, nerve cells will not be able to function normally and may die. Mitochondria are sensitive to oxidative stress.

Protein Aggregation

Proteins in cells are continually being broken down and replaced, which is the basis for the often-told story that one's body is replaced every 7 to 10 years. There are mechanisms to recycle protein parts into new proteins. If the breakdown process is impaired in upper and lower motor neurons, old proteins may not be broken down and can form clumps, or **aggregates**. Abnormal clumps may cause the formation of more aggregates, and the aggregates may be toxic to the nerve cell and contribute to cell death.

Abnormal clumps or aggregates of protein occur in many neurodegenerative diseases, including Parkinson disease and Alzheimer disease. Thus research on the pathologic role of aggregates in another disease may help our understanding of ALS.

Immune Dysfunction

The **immune system** may have a role in ALS. When cells die from any cause, the immune system helps remove them. In ALS, the immune system may become overactive and contribute to nerve cell damage.

Gene Mutations

Genes contain the code to make all of our proteins. Some patients with ALS have a clear family history linked to a **mutation** in a gene. The gene mutation results in the production of an abnormal protein or no protein. The abnormal or missing protein may lead to or contribute to motor neuron death. More information on fALS and gene mutations appears later in this chapter.

Challenging Facts about ALS

While we cannot explain why nerve cells die in ALS, a number of challenging facts must be accounted for when researchers investigate causes:

- ALS and the other neurodegenerative diseases are primarily diseases of adults and rarely begin early in life; thus aging of the nervous system is a factor. This is even true of fALS, where the faulty gene has been present from birth. Accordingly, ALS onset in the third decade of life is very rare, and the frequency increases to a maximum in the late sixth or early seventh decades (Figure 1–2). The frequency decreases in later decades, likely because more common diseases occur that are fatal.

- ALS starts with focal symptoms in one area of the body, and symptoms then spread to involve other areas of the body. This implies that the disease starts with a few neurons degenerating and dying and then spreads to involve other neurons. It is possible that the basis for this spread is that clumped or aggregated proteins from one neuron can pass the disease process to another neuron.

- There is a theory that ALS starts with degeneration of upper motor neurons, which then causes degeneration of lower motor neurons in the brainstem and spinal cord. For other forms of MND, for example, patients with primarily lower motor neuron involvement (PMA) frequently have some upper motor neuron loss at autopsy. Similarly, patients with primarily upper motor neuron involvement (PLS) do not clinically have loss of lower motor neurons, but many show a loss of lower motor neurons at autopsy.

- Some regions of the body tend to be affected earlier and more commonly than other regions. For example, in the split hand syndrome discussed in Chapter 3, muscles of the thumb and nearby fingers are affected before those on the little-finger side. In the legs, weakness frequently starts with a footdrop. The muscles in question may be particularly vulnerable because of the degree of upper motor neuron connection with the corresponding lower motor neurons.

- Conversely, some regions of the body tend to be affected much later. For example, nerves that control the muscles that move the eyes are affected only very late if at all, and nerves that control the bowel and bladder sphincters are almost never affected to the point of a patient's becoming incontinent.

Why Do I Have ALS?

"Why me?" is a key question, but there are no clear answers. Patients often ponder what triggered the onset of their ALS: was it trauma or something environmental, such as exposure to chemicals or microwaves, their particular occupation, or specific activities? The one known cause of ALS is hereditary transmission of a faulty gene, but the underlying factors that lead to neuron death in fALS are not known. It is important to know that ALS is not contagious, as there is no evidence that it passes from the patient to the patient's partner or caregiver. The spectrum of issues has been investigated, but no correlation has emerged. Several commonly considered factors are discussed below.

Environmental Factors

Epidemiology studies compare the backgrounds of ALS patients with those of matched control subjects to determine if there are environmental factors that differ between them. If a study identifies a difference, it is called an environmental **risk factor**, not a specific cause. Thus with a positive risk factor there is a higher chance of developing ALS, but it is important to understand this as only a potential risk: many people with ALS have not been exposed to the factor, and conversely, many people who have been exposed have not developed ALS. Overall, no known associations exist between the likelihood of developing ALS and where one grew up, where one lived in adult life, or whether one worked at a specific occupation.

Clusters

Clusters of ALS have been reported where it has been observed that a certain geographic area has more ALS patients than another.

When clusters are investigated by viewing larger geographic areas, there is no cluster effect. In addition, when environmental factors in the area are investigated, none have been found.

In the 1950s a cluster of cases of ALS and of ALS plus Parkinson disease and dementia was identified in Guam among the Chamorro Indians living in the Mariana Islands and in the Kii peninsula of Japan. The incidence of these diseases in those areas was about 100 cases per 100,000 people, which is 50 times more than in other parts of the world. Despite intensive scientific investigation, no underlying factor was found. Since then, the incidence of these diseases in these areas has dropped and is now closer to 2 per 100,000, the average rate in the rest of the world. The greater portion of those cases may be related to genetic mutations in the region.

Military Service

In 2008, the US Department of Veterans Affairs designated ALS as a presumptive service-connected disorder. The service connection was based on epidemiology studies showing that more veterans developed ALS than nonveterans. No single service activity or combination of activities or exposures has been implicated in this pattern, and the data suggest that it applies to veterans who served in World War II, the Korean War, the Vietnam War, and the Persian Gulf War. It is important that patients with ALS who served in the military register their diagnosis with the Veterans Administration, as service-connected benefits are broad in scope (see Chapter 16).

What Is Familial ALS?

Families who have multiple members with ALS may have a **genetic factor** that contributes to the development of ALS and that can be passed on to other family members. This is called fALS.

Our bodies are made up of millions of cells, and each cell contains a set of all of our genes. Genes are the instructions telling our bodies how to work. They guide cells during development to become nerves, muscles, bones, skin, and so forth. Within each type of cell, genes govern the making of proteins that are essential for our cells to work normally. If there is a change, called a mutation, in one of our genes, then the protein that gene should make might be made incorrectly or not at all. Sometimes, genes that make abnormal proteins can cause degeneration and death of neurons. More than 17 genes are associated with fALS (see Table 4–1). When these genes have a change or mutation in them and do not make a normal protein, ALS can result. Even though a fALS gene mutation is present at the birth of the individual, it may

TABLE 4–1 Genes with Mutations That Cause ALS

Gene	Gene Name[a]
C9orf72	Chromosome 9 open reading frame 72 (ALS + FTLD)
SOD1	Superoxide dismutase 1
TDP-43	TAR DNA-binding protein (ALS + FTLD)
FUS	FUS RNA-binding protein (fused in malignant liposarcoma)
OPTN	Optineurin
ATAXN2	Ataxin 2
ANG	Angiogenin
VCP	Valosin-containing protein
VAPB	Vesicle-associated membrane protein-associated protein B
DCTN1	Dynactin subunit 1
FIG4	FIG4 homolog, SAC1 lipid phosphatase domain containing
SETX	Senataxin
TAF15	TATA-binding protein-associated factor 2N
EWSR1	Ewing sarcoma breakpoint region 1
UBQLN2	Ubiquilin 2
SQSTM1	Sequestosome 1

[a] ALS + FTLD indicates genes associated with ALS or frontotemporal lobe dementia in the same family.

take decades to cause neuron death. In families with a mutation in ALS-associated genes, individuals may be at risk to pass on that gene change to their children.

How Is Familial ALS Passed On?

Genes are located on **chromosomes,** and every cell has two copies of each gene. This is because we receive one copy of each gene from our mother and the other copy from our father. If a mutation is present in one of the gene copies in a parent, that gene has a 50% chance of being passed on to a child. A gene mutation can result in a genetic disorder that may be passed on or inherited in several ways.

Autosomal Dominant Inheritance

In **autosomal dominant** inheritance, having a change or mutation in only one gene in a gene pair is sufficient to cause fALS. This gene change causes the protein to not be made correctly or to not be made at all. If one parent has autosomal dominant fALS, each of his or her children has a 50% chance of inheriting that gene mutation (see Figure 4–1). With autosomally dominant disease, the parent carrying the gene is usually affected by the mutation and has the disease, as will the child who receives the changed gene. However, if the disease does not start until late in life (as with ALS), the parent may die early from another cause without its being known that the parent had the gene mutation.

Autosomal Recessive Inheritance

In **autosomal recessive** inheritance, an individual must have the mutation in both copies of the gene to cause the associated disease. In autosomally recessive fALS, each parent of the person with ALS

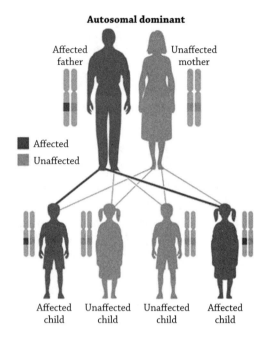

FIGURE 4-1 Autosomal dominant inheritance. One parent has a mutated gene (dark gene on chromosome) and will have the disease, and the other parent has two normal genes. Each child has a 50 percent of receiving the mutated gene from the affected parent.
Reproduced with permission from the US National Library of Medicine.

carries a change or mutation in one copy of the fALS gene and the other copy of the gene is normal. These parents are thus called carriers of the mutation. A child of two parents who are carriers of a recessive fALS gene mutation has a 25 percent, or one in four, chance of inheriting the condition (see Figure 4–2).

X-Linked Inheritance

In the **X-linked inheritance** pattern, also called sex-linked inheritance, fALS is passed to male children through their mothers. Females have two X chromosomes, and males have an X and a Y

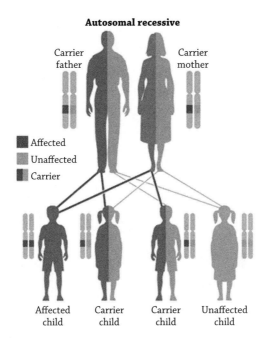

Autosomal recessive

Carrier father

Carrier mother

Affected
Unaffected
Carrier

Affected child

Carrier child

Carrier child

Unaffected child

FIGURE 4-2 Autosomal recessive inheritance. Each parent has received from his or her parents a mutation on one of the pair of genes (dark gene on one chromosome) but will not have the disease because he or she also has one normal gene. Each child has a 50 percent chance of receiving the mutated gene from each parent, but only a 25 percent chance of receiving two gene mutations (dark gene on both chromosomes) and thus having the disease.
Reproduced with permission from the US National Library of Medicine.

chromosome. A male receives his X chromosome from his mother, and his Y chromosome from his father. If a woman has a mutation in one copy of an fALS-associated gene on the X chromosome, she will not have ALS but could pass the mutation on to her children. This woman is also called a carrier. If a son inherits the X chromosome with the ALS gene mutation, he will likely develop ALS. If a son inherits the X chromosome with the unchanged or normal ALS gene, he will not develop ALS. Therefore, each son of a carrier

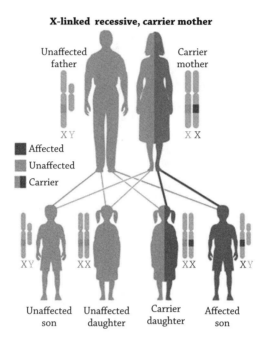

FIGURE 4-3 X-linked inheritance. Men have a single X chromosome, while women have a pair of X chromosomes. If a woman has a mutation on one X chromosome (dark gene on one chromosome), each son has a 50 percent chance of receiving the X chromosome with the mutation as his sole X chromosome (and hence of having the disease), while each daughter has a 50 percent chance of receiving the X chromosome with the mutation as one of her two X chromosomes. Like her mother, such a daughter will be unaffected but will be a carrier.
Reproduced with permission from the US National Library of Medicine.

mother has a 50 percent chance of inheriting the ALS gene mutation from his mother. Each daughter of a carrier mother also has a 50 percent chance of inheriting the ALS gene mutation but will not develop ALS, as she has a normal X chromosome from her father; however, she will be a carrier like her mother (see Figure 4–3).

In fALS, autosomal dominant inheritance is the most common pattern, autosomal recessive inheritance is very rare, and X-linked inheritance has been described in only a few families.

How Many Genes Are Associated with Familial ALS?

At this time we know of more than 17 genes associated with fALS (see Table 4–1). However, there are families with ALS who do not have mutations in any of these 17 genes. This means that other genes are associated with fALS that will eventually be discovered. Some ALS gene mutations are common and others are very rare. Interestingly, some patients with fALS have mutations in more than one ALS-associated gene.

Are There Genes Associated with Frontotemporal Lobe Dementia?

Like ALS, FTLD may be sporadic or familial. Familial FTLD is rare and follows an autosomal dominant inheritance pattern. Affected families can have members with ALS or FTLD. Thus it is important for doctors taking a family history to ask if other family members have or had ALS and if other family members have or had a dementia. One problem in reviewing a family history of FTLD is that if a family member is reported to have had a dementia, it is frequently considered to be Alzheimer-type dementia, because this is the most common type. It takes careful testing to distinguish between Alzheimer and FTLD forms, and this type of testing may not have been performed.

Are Genetic Causes of ALS and Frontotemporal Lobe Dementia Related?

Some families have members with both ALS and FTLD. The inheritance in this case follows an autosomal dominant pattern, suggesting that mutations in the same gene can cause both disorders. Several genes have been shown to cause both disorders (see Table 4–1). It is not known why the same gene mutation can affect different sets of nerve cells (those for ALS and those for FTLD).

How Do I Know If I Have Familial ALS?

The definition of "familial" when talking about inherited diseases has not been agreed upon and depends upon the inheritance pattern. In fALS, the most widely accepted definition is that ALS is familial if the patient has one or more first- or second-degree relatives with ALS (or FTLD). An example of a first-degree relative is a parent, sibling, or child. A second-degree relative may be a grandparent, grandchild, aunt, uncle, or half-sibling. The certainty of a pattern of inheritance depends upon the size of the family and how long individual members have lived. Larger families have more children and therefore greater chances of an affected child being born. Because ALS is a disease of older adults, if a family member died at a relatively young age from some other cause, he or she may not have lived sufficiently long to develop symptoms of ALS. Conversely, if an individual was very old when he or she developed ALS, the condition may not have been recognized as ALS and instead been attributed to "old age."

Another consideration is that the lifetime risk for anyone developing ALS is 1 in 350 for men and 1 in 450 for women. This means that if there are widely separated individuals with ALS in the family (not first- or second-degree relatives), it is possible that they represent two cases of sALS. It is also possible that a mutation that causes ALS occurred for the first time (and so was not inherited) in the patient being evaluated but now could be passed on from this first affected individual. As a result, there would be no family history of ALS before that individual. Overall, it is estimated that up to 20 to 25 percent of ALS patients have an underlying gene mutation contributing to their disease, and 75 to 80 percent have no genetic contribution.

Should I Have Genetic Testing for ALS?

The issue of identifying gene mutations causing or contributing to ALS is complex and is changing with new research. At this stage of our understanding, if there is no family history of ALS or dementia, there is about an 80 percent chance that the form of ALS is sporadic and will not be passed on to children. Therefore, when no family history of ALS or dementia is present, the answer to the question of whether the patient should have genetic testing for ALS is no. This is because it would be unlikely that a mutation in a gene associated with ALS would be found. Importantly, negative tests for the more than 17 known ALS-associated genes would not exclude the presence of a yet-to-be-discovered gene. Also, genetic testing for ALS is expensive.

If there is a family history of ALS, genetic testing may be worthwhile to try to determine which gene mutation is in the family. However, a family with ALS may not have a mutation in any of the known genes.

Should Family Members of Individuals with Familial ALS Have Genetic Testing?

Deciding whether family members at risk of ALS should undergo genetic testing is challenging. First, in order for the testing to be informative, a mutation in an individual affected with ALS must have been identified. Genetic testing in individuals from a family with an identified gene is becoming an important consideration, because for some gene mutations clinical trials of medications are becoming available that might slow the rate of progression of the condition. If these medication trials prove to be effective the medication might be beneficial to family members who have the mutation but who do not yet have symptoms. The role of genes in ALS is a rapidly advancing area of research. If a patient is interested in genetic testing, he or she should discuss their question with the neurologist or with a **genetic counselor**, who is a person knowledgeable about all aspects of genetics and the psychological issues of receiving a positive or a negative test result.

Chapter 5

Motor Progression in ALS

How Does ALS Progress?

Simply stated, one must expect progression. Rates of progression vary markedly among patients, from very rapid (less than 1 year from onset to death) to very slow (over many years). It is not possible to know when the first motor neuron dies, and ALS duration is measured from when the patient first recognized symptoms. Survival time for progressive and fatal diseases is commonly expressed as the median survival time (the most common disease duration). For ALS it is 2 to 4 years from symptom onset; this means that 50 percent of patients will have passed away by this time, but also that 50 percent of patients will live longer than this. The survival curve has a "long tail," and some patients have survived 10 years or more (see Figure 5–1). However, it is not possible to accurately predict at the time of diagnosis where a given patient will be on this survival curve.

We do not know why there are different rates of progression among ALS patients. Positive factors for longer survival are younger age and mostly upper motor neuron loss (patients with PLS have longer survival). Negative factors (that is, factors predicting a shorter course) have been suggested to include older age at onset and bulbar onset. However, these factors are not absolute, and many older patients with bulbar onset have slower rates of progression than younger patients with limb onset. ALS patients who also have FTLD may have a shorter time course. Every patient's ALS is different, and every patient and family feels the weakness progresses too fast!

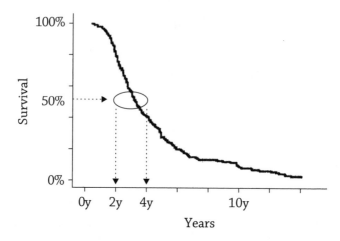

FIGURE 5-1 Survival curve for patients with ALS. Time 0y (0 years) on the horizontal axis represents symptom onset. Percentage survival is shown on the vertical axis. Median (50 percent) survival is marked with an ellipse at 2 to 4 years from symptom onset; the range is based on data from different survival studies.

The pattern of progression is for weakness to start in one place on the body, progress to involve more muscles in that region, and then progress to other regions. If the ALS starts with bulbar weakness, it is equally likely to cause weakness next in an arm or a leg. If it starts in a hand, it more likely will next affect the other hand and then the legs. If it starts in a leg, it more commonly affects the other leg and then the arms. Breathing is commonly affected midway through the course of the disease, and breathing difficulty tends to progress more slowly than limb weakness; patients may be comfortable breathing but be unable to move their arms and legs to any degree. Most, but not all, patients have difficulties with speaking, to varying degrees.

How Is Progression Measured?

ALS progression is measured in different ways in the clinic. One way is by asking the patient what has changed since the last visit, inquiring particularly about changes in function (for example, speech, swallowing, hand use, walking, and breathing). These questions are important because they allow the neurologist and others in the multidisciplinary clinic to make specific suggestions on how to manage the functional changes. The patient and caregivers are quite aware of the progression and the new challenges they are facing, hence from their standpoint, the greatest value of the multidisciplinary clinic is often the practical assistance they receive in managing the disease.

A number of measures of strength and function are described below. The results of these measures may appear in clinic summary notes available to the patient after clinic visits.

Muscle Strength

In the clinic the examiner tests individual muscles by pulling against each one. Neurologists use a simple 0 to 5 scale to rate such *static strength*, where 0 is no strength in the muscle, 5 is normal strength, and 1, 2, 3, and 4 are used for in-between levels of strength (sometimes plus and minus signs are added to the numbers for finer gradations of strength). Since muscles on one side of the body may become weak before those on the other side, one research study calculating the rate of loss of strength summed and averaged scores of all muscles tested in the arms and those in the legs. Patients were tested periodically, and when the scores were graphed against time, the loss of summed strength followed a straight line, suggesting a linear loss of strength. Rates of loss of summed strength vary among patients from rapid to slow. Measures of static muscle strength do not reflect functional or usable strength, so changes in these numbers may be useful to the doctor but are less helpful to the patient.

Functional Rating Scale

Another common way to measure progression is by using the **ALS Functional Rating Scale–Revised** (ALSFRS-R). This scale is frequently completed during clinic visits by clinic personnel. It was developed as an endpoint measure in clinical trials of potential ALS drugs (see Chapter 17). The scale assesses a patient's function within body regions: bulbar function (speech, excess saliva, swallowing), hand function (writing, handling utensils, dressing), leg function (dressing and hygiene, moving in bed, walking and climbing stairs), and breathing (shortness of breath, use of assisted breathing devices). A total score is calculated from these subscores. When total scores are plotted against time, they generally result in a fairly straight line of progression for each patient, although rates vary markedly among patients. Some patients plot their own ALSFRS-R values but may not do so accurately; regardless of accuracy, this exercise is not advised, as it does not add to the patient's sense of well-being.

How Fast Am I Progressing?

While research indicates that ALS progresses in a straight line, some patients describe an apparent acceleration of weakness, for example, rapid loss of the ability to walk. One explanation for such an apparent rapid change is that the patient was struggling with walking and was "just" able to walk, and a small additional loss of strength caused him or her to cross a threshold such that walking was no longer possible. (This is reminiscent of the expression "the straw that broke the camel's back," where just one more in a series of small weights—straws—proved too much for the proverbial animal.) Another factor is that sometimes a patient does too much in a day and may take several days to regain the prior level of strength.

> Stephen experienced greater and greater difficulty walking, and one day he just could not get out of his easy chair. He was frustrated and fearful that his ALS was taking off and progressing at an accelerated rate. His wife reminded him that he
>
> *(Continued)*

(Continued)

had been struggling to get out of the chair for several weeks, and this was the first day that he needed help. He also realized that he had been tired from walking a lot that day. The next day he managed to rise on his own, but he and his wife went to the furniture store to look for a comfortable chair with an electric lift feature.

The progressive burden of managing ALS may also cause the disease to appear to be progressing faster. Early on, the patient can manage the progression relatively easily with strategies that may include taking more time with speaking and eating, bathing and dressing at a slower pace, and walking slower and with more care. With greater degrees of weakness, basic activities require more effort, and management strategies may then include repeating words that are not understood, cutting food into smaller bites for ease of chewing and swallowing, dressing in clothes that are easier to put on and take off, and walking with a cane or walker. Another simple management strategy is trying to avoid unmanageable situations.

Lois once went into a public restroom and turned the latch on the door of the toilet stall to use the facilities. When finished, she discovered that her thumb was not strong enough to open the latch, forcing her to call out for help. Because of her voice difficulties, she must have sounded drunk, but a kind woman crawled under the stall door to unlock the latch despite being dressed in nice clothes.

At later times in the disease, even everyday activities can pose significant challenges. At this time interventions and items of durable medical equipment can be very helpful. Examples include use of communication devices if speech cannot be understood (see Chapter 11); use of a **gastric feeding tube (G-tube)** when eating becomes difficult, resulting in weight loss (a gastric feeding tube can relieve the stress of eating and lead to weight increase) (see Chapter 9); and use of a walker or wheelchair if walking becomes difficult, which reduces the number of falls and increases both safety and independence (see Chapter 12).

Does ALS Ever Get Better?

This is another commonly asked question. While there are very rare reports of patients improving, they generally fit into one of two categories. One is when a patient feels stronger for a limited time. Patients with ALS occasionally report a period of better function, and patients clearly have good and bad days. Some patients do seem to have a plateau in their progression that can last for several months. Unfortunately, it is very rare for a patient to have a sustained improvement.

The other category is descriptions on the Internet of patients being cured of ALS. These reports are difficult to objectively evaluate, because they do not include information about the initial symptoms and diagnosis. They most likely represent misdiagnoses of ALS, because if loss of lower and upper motor neurons occurs, these neurons do not regenerate and strength cannot return to normal.

Are There Staging Scales for ALS?

Patients frequently ask what stage their ALS is at. Staging scales are used for some diseases, such as cancers. In cancer, the staging describes where the cancer is located (what organ), if it has spread, and whether it is affecting other parts of the body. These factors are not issues in ALS. Staging scales for ALS are available, but they track functional changes such as when a second limb is involved or whether a patient would benefit from a gastric feeding tube or supported ventilation. Such scales are for research purposes and are not useful in the clinic or to the patient.

Chapter 6

Nonmotor Features of ALS

While ALS is considered a motor neuron disease with spasticity and weakness due to loss of upper and lower motor neurons, some patients with ALS experience a number of nonmotor features. Nonmotor features are problems that are due to degeneration of cells other than motor neurons. Examples of nonmotor features include FTLD, **emotional lability**, issues with bowel and bladder function, fatigue, change in mood, difficulties with sleep, tearing, sweating, and changes in the skin.

What Is Frontotemporal Lobe Dementia?

FTLD was introduced in Chapter 1 and will be discussed in here in detail. When one hears the term "dementia," Alzheimer-type dementia comes to mind, but there are other forms of dementia, such as FTLD. Alzheimer-type dementia is the most common form (approximately 75 percent of dementia cases), FTLD is the second most common form (approximately 15 percent), and there are a few uncommon types (approximately 10 percent). Alzheimer-type dementia is not associated with ALS, but frontotemporal lobe–type dementia occurs to varying degrees in 40 percent to 50 percent of patients with ALS. FTLD results from degeneration of nerve cells in the frontal and temporal portions of the brain (see Figure 1–1).

What Are the Features of Frontotemporal Lobe Dementia?

There are three types of FTLD: the behavioral variant, semantic dementia variant, and progressive nonfluent aphasia variant. The most common type in the setting of ALS is the behavioral variant. The features of the behavioral variant are listed in Table 6–1, but among affected patients with ALS the number of features observed and their severity vary markedly. At one extreme, which is uncommon in ALS, is a patient who presents to the neurologist with all of the symptoms to a marked degree and is given the diagnoses of FTLD. Then it is noted that he or she has muscle atrophy and weakness, and the patient is given an additional diagnosis of ALS (FTLD + ALS). It is much more common for a patient to be diagnosed with ALS and for the neurologist then to note some of the features listed in Table 6–1. When the features are mild, the patient is considered to have a frontotemporal lobe "syndrome" and not full dementia. Occasionally, the family recalls that the patient began to withdraw from social activities before weakness started. In this book, the term FTLD will be used for both full dementia and the lesser syndrome.

Why do some patients with ALS have loss of nerve cells in the frontal and temporal lobes of the brain in addition to loss of upper and lower motor neurons? And why do some patients have severe FTLD and others the less severe syndrome? These two questions have not been answered but are being studied. Interestingly, patients with other neurodegenerative disorders, such as Parkinson disease, also develop dementia many years after the start of their difficulties with movements.

How Is Frontotemporal Lobe Dementia Diagnosed?

FTLD can be diagnosed in several ways. One way is through observation of features listed in Table 6–1 during the clinic visit. For instance, the doctor may note a patient's relative indifference (asking

TABLE 6-1 Symptoms Found to Varying
Degrees in Patients with Frontotemporal
Lobe Dementia

Reduced word output

Poor quality of social interactions

Apathy

Altered emotional expressiveness

Distractibility

Irritability

Selfishness

Disinterest

Repetitive/stereotyped activities

Compulsive behaviors

Hyperorality/dietary changes

Difficulty solving problems (decision making)

---

fewer questions) when talking about the severity of ALS. When family members are queried, they may note that the patient is less outgoing and speaks fewer words than he or she used to (or is less chatty).

Another way is by administering a brief (10- to 15-minute) screening questionnaire in the clinic. The questionnaire assesses the function of the frontal and temporal lobes. A number of such screening questionnaires are available, and each clinic may use a particular one.

A third way is by administering a large battery (series) of tests to pinpoint which parts of the brain are affected. The battery is recommended when the symptoms are severe and a diagnosis of full FTLD is considered. The tests are usually administered by a **neuropsychologist** and take several hours to complete. The neurologist analyzes all the data and makes a determination of what type of dementia is present.

Brain **magnetic resonance imaging (MRI)** scans may show atrophy of the frontal and temporal lobes of the brain, but this is noted only in cases with full FTLD and not with milder forms of the syndrome.

Why Is It Important to Diagnose Frontotemporal Lobe Dementia?

It is useful to determine if a patient with ALS has elements of FTLD because it can explain certain patient behaviors observed by the family. Some behaviors can be challenging for the caregiver and family to cope with, and confirming that they are beyond the patient's control can be reassuring to the family.

> John and his wife, Carol, focused on why his hands were becoming weaker. After the diagnosis of ALS settled in, Carol noted a change in his personality. He was no longer the "can-do" guy and retreated into himself. Carol initially thought the change was due to the diagnosis of ALS, but when he became increasingly impatient with her as she had to help him more and more with his daily dressing, she began questioning her ability to be helpful. When it became apparent that his changes in personality reflected frontotemporal lobe symptoms, Carol was able not to take his negative comments about her to heart.

Difficulties with decision-making are an important element of FTLD and raise questions about whether the patient can make decisions about his or her care, safety, and well-being. For example, a patient may fall on a frequent basis because he or she does not wait for assistance walking or does not accept recommendations for walking aids and other interventions. Or a patient may put off accepting recommendations for a gastric feeding tube despite having great difficulty swallowing and losing weight as a result. The question is whether such examples are due to the patient's inability to make reasonable decisions or to the patient's expressing **autonomy** as stubbornness or not wanting to acknowledge the progressive element of ALS.

In simple situations, a family member may be able to diplomatically persuade the patient to make a "good" choice, and support from professionals at the multidisciplinary clinic can also be helpful. In complex situations, the question is whether patients with FTLD can make decisions about their safety and well-being or have sufficient understanding to participate in clinical trials and to make end-of-life choices. There is no easy answer, and one must respect patient autonomy even when a different choice seems obvious to the neurologist and family. Thus there is a gray area between autonomy and incompetence that cannot be easily clarified. Only in the most extreme cases will a family consider requesting appointment of a conservator to impose a decision on the patient, and in those cases the applicant for the conservatorship will likely be required to demonstrate that the patient is incapacitated.

How Are Symptoms of Frontotemporal Lobe Dementia Treated?

The symptoms listed in Table 6–1 vary greatly among patients. For some patients, they are mild and do not cause issues with care. For others, they interfere with care. There are no medications that are specific for FTLD. If behavior becomes an issue, a variety of medications used for psychiatric disorders can be tried, usually at low doses. It is important for the family to discuss options with the neurologist after explaining the issues. The mainstay of treatment is addressing the behavioral issues with patience, even though this can be difficult and symptoms can cause distress for the caregiver and family.

What Is Pseudobulbar Affect?

Pseudobulbar affect (PBA), also called emotional lability, is an impulse to laugh or cry that is beyond the patient's control. It occurs in varying degrees in about 50 percent of patients with ALS.

PBA also occurs in other neurologic disorders, and the nerve cells involved in causing it have not been fully identified.

What Are the Features of Pseudobulbar Affect?

The impulse to laugh or cry in PBA is usually triggered by a situation that is humorous or sad, but the magnitude of the stimulus may be mild, and the response overly vigorous. The patient usually does not feel the level of emotional involvement suggested by the vigorousness of the laughing or crying, and it may be difficult for the patient to stop laughing or crying when he or she wants to. The crying provides no cathartic relief, as emotional crying does. In the extreme, the ease of crying or laughing and difficulty stopping can prevent effective communication. Interestingly, it has been said that people with ALS seem to be very "nice." One explanation for this observation is that the ease of laughing due to PBA results in a perpetual smile that is interpreted as having a nice personality.

Another symptom that occurs in some ALS patients and is attributed to PBA is an increase in the frequency of yawning and in how wide the yawns are. The reasons why everyone yawns and why yawning can be increased in ALS are not known.

Lois became more emotional shortly following her diagnosis, and sometimes laughed or cried over things that previously would not have affected her. On one memorable occasion, the family cockatoo was flying from one person's shoulder or hand to another. Lois got the giggles and just couldn't seem to stop. Everyone laughed and enjoyed their time together even though her reaction was overly vigorous. She experienced other, similar episodes, as when relating her experience with the locked toilet stall (see Chapter 5), even though prior to the onset of ALS she would have been mortified by that experience.

How Is Pseudobulbar Affect Diagnosed?

For physicians, the presence of PBA in some patients is obvious during clinic visits. With other patients, asking the patient and family about more rare occurrences is useful. A brief questionnaire that can be administered in the clinic provides a score that helps determine if there are no symptoms, mild symptoms, or marked symptoms of PBA. The questionnaire can be used to judge the effectiveness of treatment.

Why Is It Important to Diagnose Pseudobulbar Affect?

Patients may experience sudden and uncontrollable laughing and crying in public, be embarrassed, and then not want to appear in public again. Once a diagnosis is made, the condition can be treated.

How Is Pseudobulbar Affect Treated?

The cause of PBA is not fully known, though it is associated with (but not caused by) upper motor neuron loss. It is believed to be due to changes in levels of neurotransmitters. Medications that affect neurotransmitter levels are effective in treating PBA. Two medications are available (Table 6–2): Amitriptyline (brand name Elavil) is an antidepressant that has a number of uses for treating symptoms in ALS that are independent of depression. Nuedexta is a two-drug combination of dextromethorphan and quinidine. Dextromethorphan is the active drug but is usually very rapidly degraded in the bloodstream; quinidine blocks the breakdown of dextromethorphan, allowing a sufficient amount to reach the brain.

TABLE 6–2 Medications Used to Treat Pseudobulbar Affect

Medication	How Supplied	Preparation	Crushable	Dosage	Frequency	Side Effects
Amitriptyline (Elavil)	Prescription	Tablet	Yes	25 to 50 mg	At night	Anticholinergic
Dextromethorphan/ quinidine (Nuedexta)	Prescription	Tablet	No	20/10 mg	2 times daily	

Betty was generally withdrawn, but she also had PBA. She attended the wedding of a friend's daughter and burst out laughing during the ceremony. Needless to say, she was very embarrassed and said that was the last event she would attend out of the home. This episode was discussed at the next clinic visit, and Betty was prescribed a medication that gave her more control. She was able to attend another wedding several months later without any embarrassing incidents.

Can ALS Cause Changes in Bowel and Bladder Function?

In ALS, patients do not become incontinent (lose control of their bowels or bladder), but changes in function can occur. A small percentage of patients describe urinary and occasionally bowel **urgency**. This means that they have a marked need to get to the bathroom, which they may have difficulty reaching because of leg weakness and slow walking. The cause of this urgency is not known, but it likely represents an overactive bladder or overactive colon. Normally, urgency and the ability to hold on until reaching the bathroom can be managed. We know that infants do not have control over urination or their bowels but develop such control within a few years. Thus urgency in ALS is likely due to loss of some nerve cells in the brain, but it is not known which ones are involved. A number of medications can be prescribed to reduce urinary and bowel urgency (see Chapter 13).

Some patients with ALS describe needing to empty their bladder more frequently at night, which can disturb sleep for both the patient and caregiver. It is not clear why this increase in frequency occurs. Reducing fluid intake in the late evening, except to swallow pills, is one approach to attempting to manage this symptom. Other suggestions are to use a bedside commode or, for men, a bedside urinal. Men can also benefit from use of an external or condom **catheter** at night. The patient should inform the physician if frequent urination becomes a problem, both to get a better night's sleep and also to reduce strain on the caregiver.

> Lois experienced a marked problem with urinary urgency at night. It became very burdensome for her husband, Ray, to physically get her to the bathroom numerous times during the night, particularly when there was no actual need to use the toilet. Ray's solution was to place a commode next to the bed. When Lois became so weak that she could not assist in the transfer to the commode, he also got a lower bed to reduce the strain on him from repeatedly lifting Lois in and out of bed.

Patients with ALS frequently have constipation, likely due to several factors. One factor is general inactivity from muscle weakness, which is difficult to change. Another factor is reduced fluid intake, which may result from trying to reduce the frequency of bathroom visits because of walking difficulties. A third factor is **anticholinergic side effects** of some medications given to patients with ALS to treat certain nonmotor symptoms. Medications with anticholinergic properties and options for treating constipation are discussed in Chapter 13.

Why Do I Feel So Fatigued?

Some patients with ALS note marked fatigue, even though they are physically doing less because of weakness. There are several possible reasons for this fatigue. First, even though patients are physically doing less, the weak muscles are working harder than when they were strong, and thus they are expending more energy than they used to.

Patients and their doctors focus on the obviously weak muscles during clinic examinations, but other muscles that appear "strong" on examination are actually weaker than before ALS. Thus these hard-working muscles are contributing to a greater level of fatigue. There is little that can be done to reduce fatigue from weak muscles, but understanding the underlying factors may reduce frustration.

There is a concept of "budgeting energy" in ALS, as a patient is considered to have a daily "allowance" of energy that is reduced over time as weakness progresses. Expending a large amount of the allowance early in a day will leave the patient fatigued at the end of the day. Budgeting across the day can leave some energy for activities at the end of the day, such as receiving visitors.

Another form of fatigue is called **central fatigue**. This is a feeling of tiredness that is not attributable to weak muscles or high levels of activity. It is likely due to changes in neurotransmitters, and many transmitters may be involved. Central fatigue can be exaggerated by low mood or depression. Mood-elevating medications can help, and the issue should be explored with the doctors providing care.

ALS Can Be Depressing. How Do I Know If I Am Depressed?

Both the patient's and the caregiver's moods will be affected by ALS. First there is the shock of the diagnosis, then a feeling of loss, then pulling together with family to cope with the challenges, and finally working through the final stages. Many factors can affect a person's mood. How one copes with new issues related to ALS also depends upon how one managed challenging issues in the past. Some patients have had issues with depression before ALS, and some have taken or are taking medications for mood at the time of diagnosis. The diagnosis and course of ALS may cause a preexisting depression to return or worsen.

Interestingly, depression is relatively uncommon among patients with ALS, and only about 15 percent test in the depression range on depression screening tests (with only a few of these patients testing in the very depressed range). The human spirit is very robust, and people can find meaning in the face of challenges. Some people with ALS consider it a gift, as they can focus on what is important to them and derive added meaning in their lives. They can also communicate their final messages to loved ones, since they have sufficient advance notice to do so.

A person's mood is extremely important, and many factors should be considered before a diagnosis of depression is made. One factor is fear of the future, and related to this is inaccurate information obtained from less-than-reliable sources. Thus it is essential that frank questions be asked of the neurologist and others in the multidisciplinary clinic about what will happen and when. It must also be appreciated that the neurologist may not have exact answers but should be able to give useful information. Pain is another factor that can negatively affect mood if not adequately controlled (see Chapter 13). A third factor is sleep, which may be disturbed in ALS for a number of reasons (see Chapter 13).

When all of these issues are considered, a significant percentage of ALS patients may benefit from mood-elevating medications such as **selective serotonin reuptake inhibitors (SSRIs)** (see Chapter 13). ALS can also affect a caregiver's mood, which can in turn affect the patient (see Chapter 16).

Why Have I Noticed Changes to My Skin?

It is not uncommon for patients and caregivers to comment on changes to the skin. The skin is a complex tissue and includes a set of small nerves going to sweat and tear glands. These nerves are part of the **autonomic nervous system**, or involuntary nervous system, which controls many internal bodily functions, including skin function. Although they are different from the large motor nerves that cause weakness in ALS, there are also changes in small nerves. Similar changes in the autonomic nervous system occur and have been studied in many other neurodegenerative diseases, but few studies have been performed on these changes in ALS.

Why Do I Have Scaly Skin?

The skin about the face can feel greasy or oily in ALS, and there can be flaking (dandruff) about the eyebrows and hairline. These symptoms are also due to changes in the autonomic nervous system. They can be managed by cleaning and dandruff shampoo.

Lois was so concerned about the increased dryness of her skin that she thought she was bathing too frequently and stopped bathing altogether. This concern, when combined with a mild FTLD, resulted in a marked change in her personal hygiene habits. It was not easy to persuade her that the problem was not the result of bathing too frequently. It was only after it was suggested that she take joint showers with her daughter, followed by use of a soothing lotion, that Lois agreed to resume her normal bathing schedule. Following that initial breakthrough and confirmation from the nurse at the multidisciplinary clinic that bathing was a necessary part of good hygiene, bathing was no longer an issue for Lois.

Why Do I Sweat So Much?

A small percentage of patients with ALS can have profuse sweating, usually about the face and upper body. Tearing and sweating require nerves to activate tear and sweat glands. Excessive sweating occurs when these nerves are overactive, in contrast to motor neurons in ALS, which are underactive and die. Sweating can be managed by providing a cool environment, perhaps with an airstream from a fan, and wiping away the sweat.

Why Do My Eyes Sting?

A small percentage of patients with ALS describe excess tearing and a stinging feeling in their eyes. The cause of the stinging feeling is not clearly understood, but it likely reflects irritation of the eye by excess tears (not necessarily full teardrops) and oils from the skin that reach the eyes. The stinging responds to wiping the eyes with a damp washcloth or facial tissue. Patients who have arm weakness describe stinging more often, possibly because they cannot easily wipe their eyes.

Why Do I Bite My Cheek?

A number of ALS patients mention that they bite the insides of their cheeks or their tongue more than they used to. This likely is due to either poor control of biting from upper motor neuron loss or weakness of tongue and facial muscles from lower motor neuron loss.

Why Are My Hands or Feet Red, Swollen, or Cold?

When muscles become weak in a hand or foot, less movement occurs in that part of the limb. As a result, the hand or foot may become red (even purple), puffy, and cold to the touch. Redness is due to blood pooling in the skin when the limb is not being used. Puffiness is due to decreased ability to move the normal accumulation of fluids through the **lymph system** (note that everyone's feet swell when movement is confined, as in air or car travel). Coolness is due to weak muscles not requiring as much warm blood. These changes are not due to abnormalities of blood circulation and are not harmful. They do not need to be treated with water pills, but a patient can wear compression hose or compression gloves to reduce redness and puffiness.

Do I Have to Worry about a Deep Venous Thrombosis (Blood Clot)?

A **deep venous thrombosis (DVT)** is a blood clot in a deep-lying vein. Blood clots do occur in patients with ALS, but they are rare. The redness and puffiness discussed above are due to immobility of a limb and are not due to a blood clot. If there is markedly painful swelling in the lower leg (above the ankle), thigh, or upper arm, the patient should seek medical attention promptly to determine if the pain is from a deep blood clot.

Do I Have to Worry about Skin Pressure Sores?

When people become immobile they may have breakdown of the skin from not being able to change position, leading to pressure or bedsores. Interestingly, in ALS, even when marked weakness prevents changes in body position, pressure sores are very rare. This suggests that there are changes to skin cells or cells that are just under the skin (subcutaneous tissue) unique to ALS that protect against skin breakdown. Research shows changes to collagen in the subcutaneous tissue. Nevertheless, it is important to inspect bony parts for redness and early skin breakdown in ALS patients.

Chapter 7

Management and Treatment of ALS

Care of the ALS patient can be optimized by being followed in a multidisciplinary care ALS clinic where medical personnel have experience with medications to treat and manage symptoms associated with the disease.

Do I Need a Primary Care Physician?

The answer is yes, as a **primary care physician (PCP)** is important in the care of non-neurologic issues, whether present at the time of the ALS diagnosis or developing after the diagnosis. For example, ALS is primarily a disease of older adults, and many patients will have elevated blood pressure, heart conditions, or other conditions associated with aging. The PCP is the best person to manage these conditions. Because ALS patients may develop a new medical issue during the course of ALS, the report from the ALS clinic visit should be sent to the PCP.

Should I Continue with My Current Medications?

The answer is yes, as the goal is to maintain good health even in the setting of ALS. However, there are data suggesting that elevated lipids in the blood contribute to improved longevity for ALS patients. Accordingly, in our ALS clinic we normally recommend that a patient should discuss stopping lipid-lowering medications with the PCP.

Where Can I Get the Most Comprehensive Care?

The most comprehensive care is offered in a multidisciplinary ALS clinic having a wide spectrum of healthcare providers representing many disciplines available at each clinic visit. A large number of multidisciplinary ALS clinics exist throughout the United States, usually in major medical centers, and most major university medical centers also have a multidisciplinary ALS clinic. Clinic locations in the United States can be obtained from online websites for the Amyotrophic Lateral Sclerosis Association (ALSA) or the ALS division of the Muscular Dystrophy Association (MDA).

If no multidisciplinary clinic is available, private practice neurologists can provide good care and frequently refer patients to healthcare providers in other disciplines to assist in care. Such an approach requires several clinic visits, and the other providers may not be as experienced with issues that arise in patients with ALS as are providers at multidisciplinary ALS clinics.

What Happens in a Multidisciplinary ALS Clinic?

The multidisciplinary ALS clinic has been found to be the most efficient way to provide care, and it can take 2 to 4 hours to be seen by the full range of providers in a single visit. The following sections describe core providers.

Neurologist

The neurologist is a doctor who diagnoses and treats disorders of the nervous system. Neurologists in multidisciplinary ALS clinics have a special interest in the disease and are familiar with all aspects of it. Roles served by the neurologist include making the diagnosis and answering questions about the pathology and progression of the disease. The neurologist frequently participates in clinical research trials (see Chapter 17).

Nurse

The nurse in a multidisciplinary ALS clinic is also familiar with all aspects of ALS and is the most accessible person on a day-to-day basis, available by telephone between visits to answer questions. Nurses have experience with how to manage issues and where to obtain resources.

Speech-Language Pathologist

The speech-language pathologist is familiar with managing changes in speech and swallowing that occur in ALS. The speech-language pathologist recommends communication strategies, including simple (low-tech) aids and more complex (high-tech) devices using mobile telephones, tablets, and computers. The speech-language pathologist also assesses the patient for swallowing difficulties and makes recommendations for gastric feeding tubes.

Occupational Therapist

The occupational therapist is familiar with managing changes in hand function and recommends alternative ways to carry out activities of daily living. The occupational therapist provides wrist braces or hand splints to improve dexterity and supplies aids for dressing.

Physical Therapist

The physical therapist is familiar with managing changes in leg function and walking. The physical therapist can recommend braces (**ankle-foot orthoses**, or AFOs) for footdrop; canes, walking sticks, walkers, and wheelchairs for impaired mobility; and lifts to aid transfers.

Respiratory Therapist

The respiratory therapist is familiar with managing changes in breathing function and with tests for breathing strength. The respiratory therapist recommends breathing exercises and assists with the selection and use of **noninvasive ventilation** devices.

Dietitian

The dietitian is familiar with managing weight loss. The dietitian recommends changes in diet when swallowing becomes difficult, manages nutritional formulas for patients using a gastric feeding tube, and makes suggestions for managing changes in bowel function.

Social Worker

The social worker is familiar with the emotional and family stresses associated with ALS as well as available social services. The social worker serves as a counselor for the patient, caregiver, or children; directs patients and families to social services and resources; and helps select legal documents for end-of-life care.

Genetic Counselor

In the setting of familial ALS, genetics can be complicated. The genetic counselor answers questions about inheritance, counsels on the emotional issues surrounding genetic testing, and selects laboratories for genetic testing.

Palliative Care and Hospice

ALS is progressive and shortens life. The **palliative care** team can optimize quality of life. The group includes a physician (who can be the neurologist), nurse, chaplain, and home health aides. Palliative care begins with the diagnosis of ALS. The degree of involvement is low early on and involves **hospice** care late in the course of the disease.

The following group of physicians and providers is not usually present in the ALS clinic but can be called upon when necessary.

Pulmonologist

The **pulmonologist** is a doctor trained to manage respiratory symptoms and works with the respiratory therapist. Together they manage respiratory complications related to ALS and **invasive ventilation** when a patient chooses it. They also manage other respiratory issues that may have been present before the onset of ALS (for example, emphysema, chronic obstructive pulmonary disease, or asthma).

Gastroenterologist

The **gastroenterologist** is a doctor trained to manage digestive issues. For ALS patients the gastroenterologist places a gastric feeding tube when adequate nutrition cannot be maintained by oral feedings.

Psychiatrist

The **psychiatrist** is a doctor trained to manage behavioral issues that can occur with FTLD and major mood issues. Occasionally a patient with other psychological or psychiatric diseases develops ALS, and the psychiatrist also prescribes medications for those diseases when needed.

Psychologist

The **psychologist** has a doctoral degree and functions similarly to the psychiatrist to manage issues with mood and behavior, but does not prescribe medications. The psychologist also serves as a counselor.

Orthotist

The **orthotist** is trained to evaluate gait (walking) disorders and can make recommendations for ankle braces (AFOs) and knee braces.

How Often Should I Be Seen in the Clinic?

In general, patients are seen every 3 months in a multidisciplinary clinic. From practical experience this is a good interval, allowing changes to be queried and plans to be made for the next interval. However, issues may arise between clinic visits, and it is important to contact the clinic nurse and not wait until the scheduled visit if they do. When issues cannot be addressed over the telephone, a focused clinic visit can be arranged.

Should I Attend a Support Group?

Support groups are monthly meetings for patients and caregivers put on by supporting organizations such as the MDA or the ALSA. They include one or more moderators and serve several purposes. One is to show that the patient and caregiver are not alone in what they are experiencing and that there are others who appreciate the challenges. Another is to provide advice on managing current and future issues. A third is as a source of emotional support for the patient and caregiver, as most support groups have separate sessions where the patients and the caregivers can talk among themselves. Meetings frequently have outside speakers, including neurologists who provide research updates, various therapists (speech-language pathologists, dietitians, or occupational, physical, or respiratory therapists) who make suggestions for managing activities, and others who talk about social services (Social Security and disability, veterans' benefits). Support groups give both patients and caregivers an opportunity to compare notes with other patients and caregivers, and there are times when an idea or solution discussed by a friend or someone facing a similar problem will have more impact and be more helpful than the same information imparted by a professional.

> Lois enjoyed the support group so much that she planned her periodic multidisciplinary clinic visits around the support group schedules. Since she lived over a hundred miles from the support group, Lois wanted her daughter to attend the group alone when Lois was not in town, and she was eager to hear reports about how her friends were doing. Those reports seemed more important to Lois than information about other topics presented at the meetings

Benefits of support groups vary for the patient and caregiver, and some patients and some caregivers do not feel comfortable attending them. Sometimes it is the caregiver who goes when the patient does not want to attend. In our ALS clinic we strongly urge patients and caregivers to investigate the local support group and attend at least one session.

> At their first multidisciplinary clinic visit, John and Carol were told about the local ALS support group, but John did not want to go and "see what will happen to me." Carol felt overwhelmed with John's progressive weakness and his reluctance to accept
> *(Continued)*

(Continued)

help and decided to attend alone. She found other caregivers facing similar challenges and felt better. After several months John attended a session and made friends with other patients.

What Is Available on the Internet?

The Internet is extensive, with many sources of information, some accurate and some not. There are agencies that provide reliable information, including the ALSA, MDA, and the National Institutes of Health, whose website page www.clinicaltrials.gov gives information on ALS clinical trials.

Online patient and caregiver chat rooms allow for sharing experiences. One is www.patientslikeme.com, which is an online health network that was started by a family with a member with ALS and has expanded to include many other diseases. This website allows patients to input data on their conditions; give treatment histories; discuss symptoms, treatment effects, and side effects; and list disease-specific functional scores on an ongoing basis.

The Internet also includes advertisements for treatments and "cures" for a large number of diseases, including ALS. Many of these treatment programs have limited data to support their efficacy and a high cost. ALS neurologists are open to any treatment that would be helpful, and a group of such neurologists actively investigates Internet claims of treatment successes. Its reports can be found at www.ALSUntangled.com.

What Should I Take for My ALS?

Treatments for ALS can be divided into two categories, those that modify the disease (slow the rate of progression) and those that treat symptoms associated with ALS. The first category includes medications that will be discussed in this chapter. This category also includes interventions, such as gastric feeding tubes and assists for breathing, that may slow the rate of progression; these will be reviewed in Chapters 9 and 10. The second category consists of medications that treat symptoms and will be discussed in Chapter 13.

What about Riluzole (Rilutek)?

Despite much research to find drugs or interventions that slow the progression of ALS, none so far have been found that are markedly effective. **Riluzole** (brand name **Rilutek**) is the only medication approved by the US Food and Drug Administration (FDA) for slowing the rate of progression. It was developed and tested in two drug trials, where it was shown to have a statistically significant positive effect on survival in ALS patients. Specifically, there was an approximate 9 percent benefit in survival after taking the drug for 12 months, equaling about an additional 2 to 3 months of survival. However, this effect on progression is small and cannot be detected by the patient. It is important to understand that a statistically significant effect means that the effect is likely real and not due to chance, even if the effect is small. It is uncertain whether riluzole continues to be effective after 12 months of treatment or when a patient is markedly weak. How it works is not known, but it is thought to reduce the amount of glutamate, the neurotransmitter released by each nerve impulse at upper and lower motor neurons (see Chapter 4).

Rilutek was approved in 1994 in the United States, and in June 2012 the patent expired. Since then it has been available under the generic name of riluzole. The dose is listed in Table 7–1. There is no benefit to taking a higher dose. Side effects are very few, and although liver function enzymes need to be tested every 6 months, it is rare that riluzole has to be stopped because of side effects.

TABLE 7-1 Medication Used to Treat the Course of ALS

Medication	How Supplied	Preparation	Crushable	Dosage	Frequency	Side Effects
Riluzole (Rilutek)	Prescription	Tablet	Yes	50 mg	2 times daily	Liver toxicity (must be monitored)

Not all ALS clinics recommend riluzole, because the positive effect on patient survival of approximately 9 percent is too small to be recognized by the patient, and progression of weakness will continue over time when taking riluzole. Nevertheless, given the inexorable progression of ALS, the American Academy of Neurology (AAN) and the European Academy of Neurology (EAN) recommend riluzole for ALS patients, at least early in the course of the disease. In our ALS clinic we recommend patients take riluzole because any slowing, no matter how small, is a positive factor.

What Else Is Available?

It is understandable that when the medical community cannot offer an effective therapy or a cure for ALS, patients may turn to alternative therapies. Furthermore, family members and friends may recommend alternative treatments with the thought of "Try it, what do you have to lose?" Numerous sites on the Internet list products or treatments that claim to "cure or improve" strength in ALS. The challenge with ALS is that when a nerve cell degenerates and dies, there is no way to replace it (at least at this time), and the functions are permanently lost. Thus no drug or intervention can improve lost strength caused by ALS. While the ALS medical community would welcome any new medication or intervention, claims for improving strength or function raise concern that the positive effects are overstated. It is important to note that rarely have alternative treatments been fully tested in patients with ALS to show efficacy. There is also the concern that an alternative therapy could be harmful. Before taking any alternative treatments, patients should discuss them with their neurologists to be sure of their safety. The issues around "just trying something" are also discussed in Chapter 17.

Below we discuss a number of treatments that patients commonly ask about.

What about Stem Cells for ALS?

Patients with ALS frequently ask about the use of stems cells to treat the disease. Stem cells have a promising future in medicine, but research for their use in ALS is still at an early stage. There are different types of stem cells. The original stem cell in the body is the ovum after implantation (fertilization) by the sperm, which ultimately differentiates into all organs of the body. Clinically usable stem cells come from the initial division of the fertilized ovum into about eight cells, and cells of this type are called **embryonic stem cells**. Other stem cells are available after further differentiation and include **bone marrow stem cells** and fat, or **mesenchymal, stem cells**. All stem cells can be forced in a test tube to further differentiate into cells related to the nervous system, including **glial cells** and nerve cells.

What Can Stem Cells Do?

Use of stem cells for ALS has limitations. Stem cell therapy in ALS is different from bone marrow stem cell treatment, which has cured certain cancers, in at least two ways. First, it is not possible for a stem cell to replace an upper or lower motor neuron that has died from ALS. This is due to the fact that the distance an axon (the fiber that transmits the neuronal signal) would have to travel from a stem cell neuron to the target neuron—the nerve cell the new neuron should connect to—is too long, measuring several inches to several feet. Second, because neuron death in ALS is progressive, more and more neurons will have to be replaced as time goes on.

Current research focuses on stem cells secreting chemical factors that might preserve neurons that are otherwise destined to die from ALS. These stem cells can be either glial cells or nerve cells. These cells can be programmed to secrete large amounts of **nerve growth factors**. Nerve growth factors are proteins that cells normally produce and that are most active during fetal development, when they help guide growing nerve cells to their appropriate targets. In adult brains, nerve growth factors are produced when the brain is stressed from injury, and such nerve growth factors may reduce further death of neurons. Thus in ALS, the goal is to introduce stem cells that produce large amounts of nerve growth factors to help slow the death of neurons that are degenerating. Another approach is for stem cells to modify the immune system, although the mechanism by which stem cells would have a positive effect in altering the immune system is not clear at this time. There are greater challenges to the use of stem cells to alter the course of FTLD. At this time no long-term data exist to indicate whether stem cell therapy prolongs survival in ALS.

How Are Stem Cells Delivered in ALS?

Stem cells have an innate ability to move on their own to areas of brain damage, but it is desirable to deliver stem cells more directly to the area where neurons are degenerating. To optimize this in ALS, stem cells can be placed in the cerebrospinal fluid during a lumbar puncture (spinal tap) or directly injected into the spinal cord during an extensive surgical procedure. Both routes are under investigation.

Where Can I Get Stem Cell Treatment?

At this time, formal trials of stem cell therapy in the United States are regulated by the FDA to ensure their rigor. The phases of research that ensure rigor are discussed in Chapter 17. Research on using stem cells for treating ALS is at an early stage, and the goal at this stage is to determine safety. Each stem cell study has inclusion and exclusion criteria, and patients must contact participating centers to see if they qualify to participate. Current trials and participating clinics can be found on the Internet at www.clinicaltrials.gov.

The Internet also lists commercial clinics that advertise stem cell treatment for a large number of diseases and conditions, including ALS. These commercial clinics often boast in their marketing that their stem cells will result in improved strength or even a cure. Unfortunately, these promises for ALS are not realistic. The clinics and their stem cells are not regulated by the FDA and are not held accountable for their advertised effects. Further, treatments are very expensive, costing $10,000 to $50,000 per treatment, and multiple treatments may be recommended. In contrast, the costs of formal stem cell therapy trials in the United States are covered by industry or grants and not by the patient. In our ALS clinic we discourage patients from receiving unproven stem cell treatments but are still supportive of patients who choose to receive stem cells. We also point out that the $10,000 to $50,000 spent on an unproven therapy could be used on home renovations (for example, of the bathroom) that would be appreciated by the patient many times per day.

What about Dietary Supplements and Alternative Therapies?

Dietary supplements include vitamins and natural products. It is common for people to use alternative therapies for many disorders, and a large number of ALS patients use supplements. Supplements can consist of single categories, such as proteins or vitamins, while others are formulations or a sequence of products. A few common categories are discussed below.

Will Protein Supplements Build Muscle?

It may be reasonable to think that additional protein will build up muscles that are shrinking because of ALS, but muscle atrophy is caused by loss of lower motor neurons and not lack of protein. While protein supplements will not be harmful, sufficient protein comes from food in the diet, and more will not improve strength in the ALS patient.

Can Creatine Give Me More Strength?

Creatine monohydrate is used by bodybuilders as an aid to increasing muscle energy and strength. Several drug trials of high-dose creatine given to patients with ALS did not show a positive effect on strength or longevity. Those who choose to take it should be aware that creatine absorbs water from blood, making it important to take only the recommended dose and to drink extra water when taking it.

Can Chelation Therapy Get Rid of Toxins?

Chelation means "binding to," and chelation medications are used to bind to and remove excess amounts of metals or minerals from the body. Traditional chelation therapy involves venous infusion of a drug that attaches to and removes a heavy metal (such as lead, arsenic, mercury, or thallium) from the body. The most common chelating agent is ethylenediaminetetraacetic acid (EDTA). This chelating agent has significant side effects and is recommended only when there is proven lead toxicity. While lead levels have been found to be mildly elevated in some patients with ALS, a formal trial of EDTA in patients with ALS did not result in changes to the course of the disease.

Other forms of chelation therapy, taken by mouth, are available on the Internet. Advertisements for these products are less specific regarding what they remove, referring only to "toxic substances." However, no known toxins in the body are related to ALS, and these treatments are not felt to have an effect on ALS.

Should I Replace My Amalgam (Silver) Dental Fillings?

Amalgam is an alloy of mercury (50 percent), silver (20 to 30 percent), copper (8 percent), and other metals in trace amounts. It is used for silver fillings in teeth. An increase of mercury in the body is associated with amalgam fillings, and there are neurologic disorders associated with very high levels of environmental mercury. However, no data exist to suggest that mercury from dental fillings contributes to the development of ALS. Silver fillings have been used for hundreds of years, and until new materials became available, amalgam was the most common material used. Thus many people have amalgam fillings who do not have ALS. Patients with ALS who have had amalgam replaced with gold or porcelain have not reported slowing in progression. In addition, the process of removing the amalgam briefly increases blood mercury levels.

What about Massage and Acupuncture?

Massage and other types of body manipulations relax the muscles and can make a person feel better and more relaxed. The effects likely last only hours, so such manipulations will need to be repeated. Teaching a caregiver to provide frequent massage, perhaps before bedtime, can help with sleep. Acupuncture is based on Oriental medicine principles and has been used to provide pain relief. Thus it can be used effectively in ALS if there is pain.

Should I Exercise?

Can Exercise Improve Strength?

Patients frequently ask about the role of exercise in restoring muscle bulk and strength. Muscle atrophy and weakness in ALS are due to loss of lower motor neurons. Exercising muscles cannot restore lost strength. An exercise program could result in a small improvement in strength, but performing daily activities using weak muscles involves a greater level of exertion than doing so with normal-strength muscles, so this is exercise for the ALS patient. If an exercise program is started, the small increases in muscle tone or strength last only as long as the program is continued. Once started, keeping to the program is important.

Exercise has other beneficial aspects. It represents a time to focus internally, perhaps to work through worries or problems, and a constructive way to relieve emotions. Exercise can also be a positive way to take hold of managing ALS.

If I Don't Exercise, Will I Lose Strength Faster?

Patients also frequently ask if continuing to use a weak muscle group is better than not using it; in other words, is ALS a situation of "use it or lose it"? Some patients continue to walk even when they have been having frequent falls for fear of rapidly losing the ability to walk, when they could go farther without falling if they used a walker or wheelchair. Whether or not a patient continues to use a weak muscle group (and struggles) will have no effect on the progression of weakness in ALS. In our ALS clinic we emphasize that a fall resulting in a serious injury is worse than any embarrassment or discomfort a patient might feel about being seen using a walker or wheelchair.

Can Exercise Be Harmful?

This is the opposite question to that above. While aggressive exercise will not increase muscle strength to a noticeable degree, there is no evidence that exercise increases the rate of loss of strength. It is reasonable that if exercise makes muscles sore for several days after, it would be wise to reduce the amount of exercise. Further, exercise programs may be tiring, and fatigue may prevent taking part in other activities. There will be a trade-off if exercise takes a day or so to recover from, but if exercise is enjoyable and manageable, it is not harmful to pursue.

Chapter 8

Living with ALS

While ALS is a challenging disease from every aspect, many patients reject the phrase "dying from ALS" and replace it with "living with ALS." This is not to be taken lightly, as many other chronic diseases have progressive courses. Furthermore, dying is part of living, and the diagnosis of a serious disease allows review of one's life and priorities. In the case of ALS, living with the disease may take many forms, such as rearranging priorities, taking long-planned trips, making or re-establishing connections with family and friends, and other activities on the patient's "bucket list."

What Will My Quality of Life Be?

An important question with ALS is how it affects quality of life. The answer is that in general, quality of life is good for people with ALS, even as strength and physical function decline. How can that be? It is known that when someone views another person with an infirmity (as evidenced, for example, by walking with a cane or using a wheelchair), they expect that person to have a reduced quality of life. However, when one asks the person with the infirmity about his or her quality of life, the rating is often much higher than that of the observer. The resolution to this seeming paradox lies in what is called a **response shift**, where the person with the infirmity shifts his or her expectations and derives satisfaction even if he or she cannot physically perform at a high level.

In a sense, normal aging represents a response shift! With youth come lofty goals, both social and physical. While we make every effort to achieve these, some are always left unmet. With age comes comfort with not having achieved all our goals and perhaps even the reprioritization of our goals.

Stephen had always played basketball until he faced the physical limitations from ALS. He played the game in high school and college (where he had a basketball scholarship) and continued playing in a church league every week. Although he was able to continue playing only for 9 months after being diagnosed with ALS, Stephen continued to derive enjoyment from basketball after his diagnosis by following both college and professional games on TV and was loyal to his alma mater's team no matter their season's successes or failures. In fact, he made a special trip to his alma mater to watch a home game.

Stephen's response shift demonstrated his ability to find an alternative way to continue enjoying his love of basketball. Other patients may comfortably discard prior activities rather than refocusing them.

Lois and Ray spent many pleasurable hours touring the country in their motor home prior to her diagnosis of ALS. A few months before Lois died, a family motor home trip with both daughters and the grandchildren was planned. Ray got the motor home in perfect shape, all the meals were prepared or planned, and one daughter and her family traveled to Utah from the Midwest. The day before the planned departure, Lois decided that traveling in the motor home was no longer important to her and that she didn't want to take the trip. She was comfortable just spending time with the family at home.

An individual's personality before the onset of a severe condition is an important issue in how that person deals with life's ups and downs. If a patient has been thrown off by life's challenges, he or she may have a harder time coping with ALS. However, most people come to terms with the challenges of ALS and meet them with resolve. When there are difficulties, talking to the social worker or neurologist about specific issues can be helpful.

What Can I Still Do?

The answer is "many things." ALS limits mobility, and for some people, speech may become difficult. Aids can help compensate for both these impairments. Communication devices can amplify soft speech or synthesize typed speech. Walkers and wheelchairs (both manual and power types) can help with mobility. While these aids may not allow previous levels of activity, they can expand the range of activities possible with ALS.

Patients are often conflicted about using an aid and may forgo participation in activities. For example, they may have difficulty deciding whether to use a wheelchair to travel to activities when walking is difficult or tiring or whether to use an electronic communication tablet when their speech is hard to understand. Everyone has a personal image of him- or herself, and some of us do not want to be observed using an aid. Further, using an electronic tablet to aid interchanges takes more time than ordinary speech. It is difficult for others to appreciate a person's image of him- or herself, but it may be helpful to consider aids as tools in a toolbox; they are there when needed and they don't define a person.

Sometimes patients with ALS have a reduced level or lack of interest in using aids. This may be caused by features of FTLD, because the most common feature of FTLD is apathy. It can be very frustrating for the families of patients with both ALS and FTLD when offers of interventions are not accepted. Managing features of FTLD is discussed in Chapter 6.

What Should I Do in the Time I Have, and When Should I Do It?

The term "bucket list" describes things that a person wants to do before he or she dies. Everyone has a bucket list, but no one, even a person in good health, can complete everything on it. So it is important to consider your bucket list early on and prioritize your desires.

Can I Travel?

People with ALS can travel, but there are precautions, mostly related to comfort and safety, that should be taken into consideration. Since ALS entails a progressive loss of strength, it is advisable to travel early in the course of ALS to derive maximal enjoyment. Logistics may be challenging, as handicap accommodations in restaurants, bathrooms, and places of lodging can be inconsistent and pose problems. Lodging may be listed as handicap accessible, but standards vary and it is wise to ask ahead about particulars, such as whether the bathroom doorframe is sufficiently wide to accommodate a wheelchair, whether the bathroom has a raised toilet seat and grab bars, and whether a roll-in shower is available. Note that portable grab bars with suction cups that can be affixed where needed can be included in one's travel kit to optimize safety. If the patient uses a walker or wheelchair, ask whether access to the hotel or room has ramps or an elevator and how great the distance is between the room and the car. Long-distance travel is tiring for everyone, but for patients with ALS it may be more fatiguing, especially when there are time zone changes. It is wise to include buffer days to allow recovery from the rigors of travel.

Conserving energy is important, and with air travel, requesting a wheelchair or using the electric cart provided in many airports is advised. Also ask to be notified in advance of the boarding announcement to allow for time to go to the bathroom. Boarding the plane early reduces concerns about competing with other passengers. If a flight requires two segments, try to schedule more than an hour between flights so as not to be hurried when moving from one gate to the next. If the patient has special physical needs, such as oxygen, noninvasive ventilation, or a wheelchair to check as baggage, it is wise to contact the airline in advance to enlist the help of their personnel.

When walking is even mildly impaired, our clinic recommends calling ahead and renting a wheelchair for use at the destination. A pretravel telephone call to the MDA or ALSA clinic at the destination should be considered, as clinic personnel can assist with arrangements or even loan a wheelchair in some cases.

Safety is a major consideration. Fatigued muscles can increase the risk of falls. Sightseeing diverts one's attention from watching where one is stepping and can lead to a misstep. If walking is becoming difficult at home, using a walking stick and a wheelchair on a trip will further reduce the risk of falling and fatigue.

Stephen and his wife, Rachel, went on a cruise to celebrate their 40th wedding anniversary and to decompress after receiving the diagnosis of ALS. The cruise went well, but Stephen tired easily on the shore excursions and even sat on the ship during some of them. Two months later, when they planned a trip to Walt Disney World with their children and grandchildren, they rented a wheelchair, and Stephen was able to participate in the activities all day. As a side benefit, he and the family had accelerated access to the rides. In retrospect, he wished that he had considered a wheelchair on the cruise.

Can I Still Have Intimacy?

Intimacy covers a broad spectrum of emotions and physical (including sexual) activities. The answer across the spectrum is yes. While the complete spectrum is important, emotional intimacy is perhaps the most important aspect for a patient with ALS and can include a large number of people in the patient's life. ALS is connected with a wide range of emotions, which can change over time. A patient with ALS can have feelings of being alone and isolated. Increasing the emotional connection with family members can reduce these feelings.

Romantic or sexual intimacy is a powerful way to be connected. Patients may feel that changes in their bodies due to ALS make them less desirable, but sexual activity does not need to stop. Over time, there may be physical limitations, but accommodations can be made. There are physical therapists in rehabilitation centers who have experience with the mechanics of sexual activity when individuals have limitations of strength and movement, and their services should be requested.

Can I Have a Child?

The answer is yes, as ALS has no effect on conception. Men with ALS have no loss of potency and have fathered babies. Women have become pregnant and carried babies to full term without issues, although if a woman is sufficiently weak from ALS that walking is difficult, the progression of ALS and the extra weight of pregnancy may make walking and mobility more challenging. Also, weakness may make delivery harder. In our clinic we recommend consultation with an obstetrician with expertise in "high-risk" pregnancies. Arm and hand weakness can make care of an infant an issue. There are no reasons not to breastfeed, and ALS cannot be transmitted through breast milk.

What Is My Legacy to My Family?

Everyone wants to be remembered. A legacy to the family can take many forms. One way to preserve your legacy is to tell your life's stories. This can be done by dictating them into a tape recorder or into a computer with voice recognition software that transcribes the oral stories into text. Most patients with ALS have grown children, and many also have grandchildren, who will treasure the stories. Patients who have young children may want to leave both stories and gifts to be opened when certain milestones are reached in the child's life, such as birthdays, marriage, or the births of the next generation's children. Messages, stories, and gifts can create distinct memories, and photographs can be put into albums to allow loved ones to reflect on past events and gatherings.

Chapter 9

Nutrition and ALS

Why Is Nutrition Important in ALS?

Nutrition plays an important role in the management of ALS. Research indicates that ALS patients who maintain their weight live longer than those who lose weight. Furthermore, patients who are well nourished are better able to recover from random medical conditions unrelated to ALS, such as a cold or flu.

All cells in the body require energy, which comes from food, and it is desirable for patients to focus on maintaining their weight. The fact is that weight gain happens when more food is eaten than burned, stable weight occurs when the same amount of food is eaten as is burned, and weight loss happens when less food is eaten than is burned, causing the body to consume itself to get the necessary extra fuel. While patients may like the idea of losing inches around their waists, it is important to appreciate that when the body loses weight, both fat and protein are burned. Since muscles are made up almost entirely of protein, the body burns muscle when not enough calories are taken in! Some ALS patients are in a hypermetabolic state and burn more calories than usual. In our ALS clinic we focus on causes of progressive weight loss and make suggestions for maintaining weight.

Why Do I Lose Weight?

Weight loss in ALS is common for several reasons. When swallowing becomes difficult, patients tire while eating because they have to chew food more and require multiple swallows to clear a mouthful. As a result, many patients tend to stop before eating a full meal. Patients with hand and arm weakness get tired from bringing food to their mouth. While the amount left behind on the plate may be small, as little as several bites, it adds up with each meal and day by day: 100 kilocalories less food per day leads to a loss of about 0.5 to 1 pound per week. (In nutrition, kilocalories are usually referred to as just "calories," and we will follow that practice in the rest of this chapter.) There may be a small reduction of muscle mass due to loss of lower motor neurons, but this form of muscle atrophy is thought to be a small contribution to weight loss in ALS. Some patients describe a loss of appetite. This is usually temporary and rarely associated with significant weight loss.

Which Foods Are Harder or Easier to Swallow?

Early problems with swallowing in ALS are the need to swallow multiple times to clear food and liquids and the tendency to choke easily. Swallowing requires the complex coordination of many muscles across several phases, starting with the tongue in the oral phase and followed by muscles in the throat during the pharyngeal and esophageal phases, where food and liquids are moved into the stomach. The oral phase is voluntary, while the pharyngeal and esophageal phases follow automatically. All the phases are affected by loss of upper and lower motor neurons. When swallowing becomes uncoordinated in ALS, some foods and liquids are more difficult to swallow, while others are easier (see Table 9–1).

Liquids are the hardest to swallow, because they travel through all the phases quickly; thus muscles have to rapidly contract, which is difficult in ALS. Swallowing pills is also hard, because muscles have to coordinate the rapid movement of water with the slower movement of pills, and the pills may get stuck along the way. Chunky

TABLE 9-1 Foods to Avoid and to Consider When There Are Difficulties Swallowing

---

Foods to Avoid
- Crumbly foods
- Seeds and nuts
- Crackers
- Popcorn
- Potato chips
- Raw vegetables
- Thin soups and broths
- Chunky-style soups

Foods to Consider

Moist/soft foods, such as
- Mashed potatoes
- Pasta
- Creamy soups
- Yogurt, custard, and pudding

---

foods and those composed of small bits and pieces are also difficult because of the possibility of getting lodged in the throat. Softer foods are the easiest.

How Much Weight Loss Is Too Much?

There is no clear answer to the question of how much weight loss is too much. In ALS, continued loss of weight between clinic visits is a concern. Few people in good health lose more than 10 pounds and maintain the new weight over time. Accordingly, continued weight loss in an ALS patient of more than 10 pounds over 6 months, particularly when there are difficulties with swallowing or fatigue with eating, is an important issue to address in the clinic.

Weight varies with a person's stature. One measure that takes into consideration a person's build is **body mass index (BMI).**

BMI equals weight in kilograms (1 kg = 2.2 lb.) divided by height in meters squared (m²; 1 m = 39.37 inches). Weight and BMI are obtained in the clinic, and websites facilitate calculations with height in inches and weight in pounds (search the Internet for "BMI calculator"). The following are guidelines for healthy and unhealthy BMIs:

- Underweight = BMI less than 18.5
- Normal weight = BMI of 18.5 to 24.9
- Overweight = BMI greater than 25

How Do I Stop Weight Loss?

Since weight loss indicates insufficient consumption of calories, increasing caloric intake is the only solution. This can be accomplished in stages: first, by enhancing the diet, and then, if that is not successful, by use of a gastric feeding tube. The clinic dietitian helps patients manage weight loss.

High-Calorie Foods

The average diet that maintains weight contains approximately 1,800 calories for women and approximately 2,200 calories for men. Among the three food groups in the diet, fats (lipids) have the most calories per gram (9 calories per gram), while carbohydrates have 4 calories per gram and proteins have 4 calories per gram. Caloric intake can be increased by focusing on high-calorie foods in the diet, adding high-calorie supplements between meals, and providing an alternate route for nutrition (a gastric feeding tube).

Adding fats in the form of butter, whole milk (or even half and half), and ice cream can enhance caloric intake in a normal diet without increasing the volume of the diet, which is important when there are difficulties with swallowing. This may be one situation where a patient can finally eat favorite high-calorie foods that were previously bumped off the menu. There may be other foods that the patient avoided for medical reasons that can now be added back into the diet. For example, a patient with high cholesterol may resume eating eggs and other foods that he or she previously avoided to keep high cholesterol in check. High cholesterol is no longer a primary concern in ALS, because research supports high levels of cholesterol and other lipids in the blood as being an advantage for longevity in ALS.

Supplements

If it becomes difficult to eat sufficient calories in meals, supplements can be considered. High-calorie supplement drinks are enhanced with lipids and have 220 to 350 calories per 8 ounces. Alternatively, caregivers can make their own high-calorie shakes or smoothies by combining high-calorie dairy products (whole milk, half and half, ice cream) and fruit.

A common question is whether protein-rich supplements can reverse loss of muscle mass in ALS. The answer is no, as discussed in Chapter 7. Extra protein in the diet does not go directly to muscle. Even outside of the ALS context, protein has few calories per gram, and adding muscle mass would take a large amount of protein supplementation. Commercial supplements for ALS are balanced with respect to lipid, carbohydrate, and protein needs.

What Is Patient-Caregiver Stress over Food?

When patients lose weight, caregivers try to prepare their favorite dishes, encourage them to finish meals, and attempt to extend their mealtimes after others have finished eating. Sometimes meals take twice the usual time. Family members also become concerned when the patient chokes while eating. The patient is doing all he or she can to eat, but it can be very fatiguing. All of this results in stress over meals between the patient and caregiver. When a gastric feeding tube is placed to ensure adequate nutrition, many patients and families feel a marked reduction in stress. In our ALS clinic, when patients indicate conflicts at meal time, we suggest that placement of a feeding tube may be beneficial for all involved.

What If I Can't Maintain My Weight despite Supplements?

When ALS patients continue to lose weight despite use of supplements, it is appropriate to consider an alternative means of getting adequate calories and fluids into the stomach. A tube can be placed that goes through the abdominal wall and ends in the stomach (gastric feeding tube, or G-tube) or, occasionally, in the first portion of the small intestines, the jejunum (**J-tube).** Feeding tubes allow patients to eat as much, or as little, as they wish and then receive the remaining necessary calories through the tube without expending time and energy taking them in by mouth. Thus a gastric feeding tube can be considered a tool to be used when needed.

Feeding tubes are all but invisible to onlookers (Figure 9–1). The tube exits the body just under the ribcage on the left side. The standard tube extends approximately 12 inches from the body, is taped across the body to prevent it from dangling, and thus is fully covered by a person's clothing. For patients concerned about having a long tube, the standard tube can be replaced with a low-profile tube after the incision has healed. The site where the feeding tube leaves the body is easy to care for; one can shower with it, and the exit site is usually covered with a gauze square with a keyhole cut in it to go around the tube.

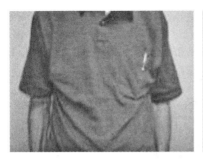
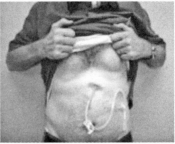
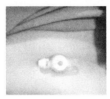

FIGURE 9-1 Patients with gastric feeding tubes. Top left: Shirt covers feeding tube, which thus is not visible. Top right: Shirt pulled up to show feeding tube. Bottom: Low-profile tube.
Photographs reproduced with permission of the patients.

How Are Feeding Tubes Placed?

A gastric feeding tube is placed in the stomach during a simple procedure. There are three types of procedures to place the tube: **endoscopy**, radiographic viewing, and surgery. The choice of which procedure to use is made by the neurologist, and factors include whether the stomach has been damaged by severe ulcers or previous gastric surgery.

Percutaneous Endoscopic Gastrostomy

Percutaneous endoscopic gastrostomy (PEG) is the most common procedure. Endoscopy refers to using a flexible scope, identical to that used to assess for ulcers, to look in the stomach. The procedure is performed by a gastroenterologist while the patient is sedated. When a suitable site in the stomach has been viewed using the endoscope, a local anesthetic is given to the skin, a small opening (approximately 2 to 3 centimeters, or 1 inch) is made in the skin and stomach, just below the ribcage, and the feeding tube is passed through the opening.

Radiologically Inserted Gastrostomy

Radiologically inserted gastrostomy (RIG) is similar to PEG placement, but the stomach is visualized by X-rays (**fluoroscopy**). The procedure is performed by an interventional radiologist. Patients are also sedated during this procedure, and tube placement is similar to that for PEG.

Surgically Placed Gastrostomy

During surgically placed gastrostomy, the feeding tube is placed by **laparoscopy** (a procedure using a fiber-optic scope looking in the abdomen). The procedure is performed by a surgeon. Patients may be sedated or anesthetized. The tube placement is similar to that for PEG.

All three of these procedures take about an hour. The risks are similar for each and include a small chance of bleeding and infection. Reduced breathing function due to ALS can be an issue for surgery, and diaphragm muscle strength is a factor when considering placement of a feeding tube. We encourage patients to have feeding tubes placed before breathing effort is less than 50 percent of predicted (see Chapter 10). Some gastroenterologists can perform feeding tube placement with breathing support using noninvasive ventilation during the procedure.

How Do I Use a Feeding Tube?

The feeding tube is easy to use to administer feedings. The end of the feeding tube has a cap, which is removed. A large syringe

(60 milliliters [mL], or 2 ounces) filled with water is used to flush out the tube and to give fluids to the patient. Nutrition is usually from commercial products called enteral formulas (available from home health companies), which vary in caloric content and other properties, but all formulas are complete with needed nutriments, vitamins, and minerals. It is also possible for a family to make food for tube feeding by blending it in a blender to allow it to pass easily through the tube, although it is time-consuming to prepare on a regular basis. It is important to be sure that blenderized food has sufficient calories and a complete range of vitamins, minerals and fiber. The advantages and disadvantages of commercial and home-blended food can be reviewed with the dietitian, who will also calculate how many calories the patient needs and will monitor weight over time, making adjustments in the number of calories as necessary.

Generally, patients take three feedings per day, with one to two 8-ounce (240 mL) cans per feeding (depending upon caloric needs). There are three methods for administering the formula: bolus, gravity, and continuous feeding. With bolus feeding, the formula is poured into the feeding tube slowly using the 60-mL syringe, and each feeding takes about 20 minutes. With gravity feeding, the formula is poured into a bag, which is hung from a support higher than the stomach, and the fluid drips in over 30 to 40 minutes. Gravity feeding is used when a patient feels bloated with the more rapid bolus feeding. Continuous feeding is given slowly, over several hours, using a pump. Continuous feeding is also used when gravity feeding is too fast or when the patient has a J-tube. Each method can be discussed with the dietitian.

Patients generally do not report feelings of hunger between meals. Occasionally, patients experience gastrointestinal discomfort, which can be managed by changes in formula or methods of delivery. The feeding tube is also good for patients who have difficulty swallowing liquids for fluid needs, and giving several large syringes of water with each feeding allows for adequate hydration.

Feeding tube maintenance is straightforward. Before and after a feeding or administration of medications, the tube is flushed with 60 mL of water. The site where the tube leaves the body requires only routine hygiene, with gentle washing with soap and water. Standard feeding tubes need to be replaced every 6 to 12 months, and low-profile tubes every 3 to 4 months. Replacement of feeding tubes is performed by the gastroenterologist.

How Do I Take My Medications If I Have a Feeding Tube?

If the patient can no longer swallow medications (pills and capsules), the clinic nurse or a pharmacist can determine which ones can be crushed and given through the feeding tube. For medications that cannot be crushed, some may be changed to liquid formulations, or changes can be made to equally effective but crushable types of medication. Medications that can be crushed or come in liquid form are reviewed in the medication tables in Chapter 13.

What Can I Expect from a Feeding Tube?

A home health company will need to be contacted prior to feeding tube placement. The clinic should arrange for a home health nurse to make a home visit 24 to 48 hours after the placement procedure to verify that feedings can be started and to instruct the patient and family on how to manage feedings. The company will arrange to supply formula, and other supplies if needed, on a monthly basis. They will make any changes based on the dietitian's recommendations.

After getting a feeding tube, patients may feel they have more energy from the better nutrition and feel less tired from the efforts of eating. And they may be reassured that they are getting the optimal nutrition for their health. Importantly, pressure to eat enough is no longer an issue. Many patients and families feel much relieved when this pressure is eliminated!

Can I Still Eat If I Have a Feeding Tube?

The gastric feeding tube does not prevent eating and drinking by mouth. A patient can enjoy bites and sips and participate in family meals. The gastric feeding tube can be considered a tool and does not need to be used all the time. In fact, there is an argument for having it placed before it is truly needed, and then it will be there when that time comes. If the feeding tube is not used for nutrition, it needs to be flushed daily with water.

Betty began her ALS with difficulties swallowing and started losing weight early on. Her husband, Henry, took over cooking and worked to make her favorite dishes, but she could not finish them because of fatigue and choking. Henry then tried supplement drinks, but they also were difficult for her to finish. Mealtimes became tense and long. Betty did not want a feeding tube, but eventually she agreed to get one. The procedure went smoothly, and she and Henry celebrated by going out to dinner with their children, with Betty taking small bites from everyone's plate. No one could see that she had a feeding tube. She then got her calories when they returned home.

Chapter 10

Breathing and ALS

How Does ALS Affect Breathing?

Before receiving the diagnosis of ALS, patients take breathing for granted. ALS rarely affects breathing as the first symptom, but as ALS progresses breathing will be impaired. Respiratory failure is the predicted cause of death in ALS, but interventions can be helpful, and a patient can even choose to prolong his or her life beyond the natural course of ALS with mechanical ventilation, as discussed below.

ALS affects breathing in two ways. The most noticeable effect is labored breathing from loss of lower motor neurons going to the diaphragm. In addition, the loss of upper motor neurons reduces the brain's control of automatic breathing. This impact is usually subtle and occurs during sleep.

How Does the Diaphragm Work?

The **diaphragm** is a thin muscle that separates the chest from the abdomen and is the main muscle used for breathing (Figure 10–1). The diaphragm is actually two muscles that work together: a right hemidiaphragm and a left hemidiaphragm, each innervated by a **phrenic nerve** (the lower motor neuron to the diaphragm). The role of the diaphragm is to move air into the lungs. In addition, **accessory muscles of respiration** raise the shoulders to help expand the chest and are activated when one is breathing hard (as after running

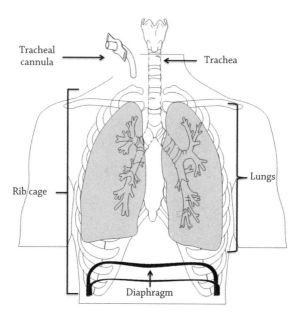

FIGURE 10-1 Diagram of the ribcage, diaphragm, lungs, and trachea. The diaphragm moves down during inhalation (as indicated by the lower of the two curves indicating the diaphragm). The trachea brings air to all portions of the lungs. A cannula may be inserted into the trachea (tracheostomy) for use with invasive ventilation.

a race) or when the diaphragm is very weak (as in ALS). Breathing in (inhalation) requires contraction of the diaphragm, while breathing out (exhalation) is passive, as air leaves the lungs without muscular effort.

The lungs are divided into right and left lobes. Air passes in and out of the lungs through the **trachea** (windpipe), which is connected to the **larynx**, which in turn connects to the mouth (Figure 10-1). The main function of the lungs is to exchange oxygen and **carbon dioxide** between air in the lungs and the blood. In the lungs, oxygen is extracted from inhaled air, and carbon dioxide is given off into exhaled air. All cells of the body need oxygen for energy production and give off carbon dioxide as the waste product. Inhaled air has approximately 21 percent oxygen and almost no carbon dioxide; exhaled air has approximately 16 percent oxygen and approximately 4 percent carbon dioxide. Breathing rate and depth of breathing are tightly regulated based on physiologic demands: they are increased during activity, when cells need more oxygen and produce more carbon dioxide, and decreased at rest.

Normal changes in breathing occur during sleep that can affect the patient with ALS. Everyone alternates between two patterns of sleep: slow-wave sleep and **rapid eye movement (REM) sleep.** During REM sleep, all muscles other than the diaphragm and those that move the eyes are effectively paralyzed, and contraction of the diaphragm becomes irregular, with brief halts in breathing. These irregularities and halts during REM sleep can be exaggerated with loss of upper and lower motor neurons in ALS and can contribute to poor sleep and a feeling of sleepiness during the day. This is why early signs of breathing difficulties in ALS frequently occur at night during REM sleep. Doctors ask detailed questions about sleep to explore whether the patient will benefit from noninvasive ventilation at night.

How Will I Know If My Breathing Is Affected?

With progressive loss of lower motor neurons to the diaphragm, the ability to breathe harder or deeper (called breathing reserve) is compromised, and patients may feel short of breath with exertion. Before that happens, patients may note that their cough, sneeze or ability to blow their nose is less forceful or that breathing may be harder when they are lying on their back (supine). One of the questions asked during clinic visits will likely be whether the patient experiences shortness of breath in bed when lying on their back; this discomfort is called **orthopnea.**

Quiet breathing is regular, but breathing becomes irregular when talking and to a lesser extent when eating. To complete a long sentence, breathing is stretched out. When breathing reserve is compromised, as in ALS, patients feel out of breath when talking and adjust by speaking in shorter sentences. The patient's speech will also be softer and lower in volume. Some patients may note shortness of breath when eating.

What Does High Carbon Dioxide Do?

Carbon dioxide is the waste product of cell metabolism and is exhaled when breathing. It is normally kept to low levels in the blood by automatic adjustments to breathing. For example, elevated levels of carbon dioxide in the blood are normally lowered by increasing the rate of breathing, but if breathing is reduced by diaphragm weakness, carbon dioxide levels in the blood rise. This can occur during sleep in the ALS patient, and the higher carbon dioxide levels can cause confusion and clouded thinking. In this case the only way to keep carbon dioxide levels in the normal range is to move more air in and out of the lungs by some form of assisted breathing.

How Is Breathing Measured in the Clinic?

Breathing is usually measured during ALS clinic visits. The most common measure is **forced vital capacity (FVC)**. FVC is the maximal amount of air that an individual can take in and exhale. To measure FVC, the patient takes in the deepest breath possible, puts in a mouthpiece that is connected by a tube to a machine, and then blows out as hard, as fast, and as much as possible. While it sounds easy to take in a deep breath, hold it, insert the tube mouthpiece, and blow, it may not be possible for patients with bulbar symptoms to coordinate these maneuvers, and a mask can be used to reduce the need for coordination. The effort should be maximal, and taking in the fullest breath and emptying the lungs completely can be a little uncomfortable, but a little discomfort ensures the best results. The volume of air exhaled is measured by the machine and expressed in liters. People of different sizes exhale different volumes of air, and the FVC result is written as "percent of predicted" based on samples taken from healthy people of the same sex, age, and height. Values more than 80 percent of predicted are considered within the normal range. Instead of blowing out as fast as possible, which can be difficult for patients with ALS, the FVC can be measured by blowing out slowly, in which case the measure is called slow FVC.

Another measure of diaphragm strength is **maximum inspiratory pressure (MIP)** or **maximum inspiratory force (MIF)**. The patient draws in the deepest breath against a closed tube, creating a vacuum, and the negative pressure is measured as centimeters (cm) of water. Values of more than –60 cm of water (that is, values of –61 cm, –62 cm, etc.) are considered within the normal range. A variation is sniff nasal inspiratory pressure (SNIP). The SNIP test is performed by plugging one nostril and inserting a tube with a seal into the other nostril. The patient is then asked to exert a maximal sniff. The tube is connected to a gauge, and normal pressures are again more than –60 cm of water.

Oxygen concentration in the blood can be easily measured with a clip on the finger by **oximetry**. This is recorded routinely in the clinic and expressed as a percentage, with values greater than 94 percent considered normal. The breathing tests described above are performed in the clinic during the day while the patient is awake and can miss early changes to breathing during sleep. Oxygen concentration can be measured in the patient's home during sleep; this is called nocturnal oximetry. The overnight tracing includes oxygen concentration and heart rate. Dips in oxygen levels associated with increases in heart rate suggest arousals (partial awakenings, of which the patient may not be aware) during REM sleep. Arousals can have different causes, but they suggest a problem with breathing during sleep that needs to be investigated further.

Carbon dioxide levels in the blood are usually more important than oxygen levels but for technical reasons cannot be easily measured in the clinic or at home during sleep. If oxygen levels from nocturnal oximetry are found to dip, it is assumed that carbon dioxide levels are elevated.

What Can I Do to Help My Breathing on My Own?

Patients can improve their breathing in a number of ways, especially during sleep. An obvious intervention is to add an extra pillow if shortness of breath occurs while lying on the back. Occasionally, patients may be more comfortable sleeping in a recliner, but this removes the patient from the bed partner, with an accompanying loss of normal intimacy. A hospital bed is a better alternative, although adjustments to the bed for patient comfort may not suit the bed partner (separately adjustable beds are available but may not be covered by insurance).

What Is Air or Breath Stacking?

During quiet normal breathing only a small percentage of lung volume is used, and some regions of the lung are minimally or not involved and are not fully aerated. Normally the lungs become fully aerated with deep breathing from general activities. If the diaphragm is weak from ALS, poorly aerated portions of the lung cannot be easily expanded with deep breaths and may collapse, resulting in reduced gas exchange. This condition is called **atelectasis**. Atelectasis can be reduced in ALS by special efforts or by noninvasive ventilation.

The technique of **air stacking** (or **breath stacking**) is one way to reduce atelectasis. It is performed by taking in a small breath, holding it and taking in another small breath, holding it and taking in another, and repeating until the last stacked breath is a supermaximal inhalation. Performing breath stacking about five times in a session (with a minute in between) in the morning and at night can help open the lungs.

Should I Stop Smoking?

Smoking can damage the air sacs in the lungs, thus reducing the ability to exchange oxygen and carbon dioxide. This is referred to as **emphysema**. It is important to appreciate that continuing to smoke in the setting of ALS is problematic. Patients are advised to stop smoking.

What Will Supplemental Oxygen Do?

If oxygen levels drop during sleep (as measured by nocturnal oximetry), patients and medical providers not familiar with ALS sometimes conclude that supplemental oxygen will help. However, supplemental oxygen rarely helps an ALS patient with breathing distress, because reduced oxygen percentage is associated with an elevated carbon dioxide level, which leads to the feeling of shortness of breath. There is usually more than sufficient oxygen in the blood even if the percentage is reduced, and supplemental oxygen will not lower carbon dioxide levels. The most effective option is to assist breathing at night through mechanical intervention, as greater air into and out of the lungs with assisted breathing both increases oxygen and reduces carbon dioxide. If a patient has both lung disease (emphysema) and ALS it is important to discuss these issues with a pulmonologist.

What Breathing Numbers Concern Doctors?

The values obtained from breathing tests administered during clinic visits are only approximations and are dependent upon several factors. If a neurologist has concerns about breathing, nocturnal oximetry may be ordered, or occasionally a full sleep study (**polysomnogram**).

Critical breathing values have not been established for ALS, but doctors begin to talk to patients about using noninvasive ventilation when one or more of the following values are recorded:

- FVC less than 50 percent
- MIP or MIF less than –60 cm of water
- Episodes of low oxygen saturation (less than 80 percent) totaling more than 5 minutes measured by nocturnal oximetry

A patient's breathing symptoms are also very important to consider, even if test numbers are in the normal range. Additional information about breathing comes from answers to these questions:

- Do you have shortness of breath during activities and talking?
- Do you need more than two pillows or are you unable to lie flat to sleep?
- Do you have morning headaches?
- Do you feel less rested after sleep than you used to?
- Are you unable to stay awake in the evening?

Why Is My Cough Weak?

A strong cough requires an extra respiratory effort, even beyond that needed for a deep breath. There are two types of coughs: reflexive, to dislodge something caught in the respiratory system, and voluntary, which can also be used when reflexive coughs are not sufficient to clear secretions. Both types of coughs require a deep inhalation, followed by a closing off of the throat, and then a forced exhalation that results in a violent rush of air when the throat is opened. The sound of the air rush in a powerful cough is like the bark of a dog.

When the diaphragm becomes weak, less air is brought in, and when the other muscles in the chest wall become weak, inhaled air is less compressed. The result is a less forceful cough, and the sound is more of a huff. A reflexive cough may be more powerful than a voluntary cough, which means that it may not be possible for a patient to voluntarily clear his or her throat when it feels like something is there, usually saliva or liquids that have not been fully swallowed because of swallowing difficulties. Continued voluntary coughing is tiring, and a patient can become very fatigued under these circumstances. In this case, the patient may try a **CoughAssist device.**

What Is a CoughAssist Device?

A CoughAssist device is a machine that helps to increase the force of a cough. When a patient wants to cough, he or she turns on the CoughAssist device, places a mask over the mouth while taking in a deep breath, and the machine provides a flow of air that is greater than the patient could take in alone. Then, as the patient starts to build up pressure and opens the throat, the machine switches to a vacuum and helps pull out the air. Another name for the machine is an insufflator-exsufflator. Patients with ALS can use it when they have difficulty clearing secretions, but they derive maximal benefit if they use it two times a day, with each use consisting of a set of three to four coughs repeated three to four times, with half to a minute or so between coughs. In our ALS clinic we introduce the CoughAssist device when the patient describes having a weak cough.

What Causes My Throat to Tighten and Make It Hard to Breathe?

Patients will occasionally feel a sudden shortness of breath and tightness in their throats that is not related to food being stuck.

There may be a harsh noise when breathing, called stridor. These symptoms, called **laryngeal spasm**, or laryngeal stridor, are likely due to the vocal cords in the larynx tightening and markedly reducing the flow of air past them. The first episode is the scariest one. It is not known what triggers the episodes, but they generally last only a few minutes. The best way to treat laryngeal spasm is to relax the vocal cords by breathing as slowly as possible; breathing fast causes more spasm. Breathing through the nose is better than breathing through the mouth for accomplishing this.

What Happens When My Breathing Becomes Weaker?

Breathing numbers obtained at clinic visits fall as ALS progresses, and patients frequently describe respiratory difficulty during sleep. When the breathing numbers or breathing symptoms described above are reached, the neurologist or respiratory therapist will recommend assisted (noninvasive) mechanical ventilation for use at night. With further ALS progression some patients will need to use noninvasive ventilation during the day, and a few will also need to use it 24 hours a day, 7 days a week. Some patients may experience acute shortness of breath due to a temporary blockage in an air passage to a section of a lung or due to pneumonia. Under these circumstances, patients may be urgently placed on a mechanical ventilator.

What Are Mechanical Aids to Breathing?

Breathing can be aided in ALS by using a mechanical ventilator. There are different kinds of ventilators, but all supply air under pressure to the patient. The air can be given to the patient in a noninvasive manner, using a mask over the nose, over the nose and mouth, or just under the nose (nasal pillows). Air can also be given in an invasive manner, using either a tube that is temporarily inserted through the mouth and into the trachea (**endotracheal tube**) or a tube that is permanently inserted directly into the trachea during a **tracheostomy** (**tracheal tube**). With noninvasive ventilation, pressure is presented at two levels, low when the patient exhales and high when the patient inhales; this approach is thus called bilevel ventilation. Bilevel ventilation is usually started at night but can be used during the day. Although bilevel ventilation at night is usually used to improve sleep, night-time use may also prolong survival. As patients continue to lose breathing strength, noninvasive ventilation can be used 24 hours a day, 7 days a week. With further progression of ALS the diaphragm becomes weaker and patients will become totally dependent upon the ventilator.

A small group of patients experience sudden shortness of breath and are treated by emergency services (the emergency department); these patients may be started on invasive ventilation. When patients are placed on a ventilator in an emergency, if the block or pneumonia cannot be resolved, the patient will need invasive ventilation 24 hours a day, 7 days a week.

A patient who uses either noninvasive or invasive ventilation 24 hours a day, 7 seven days a week, will become totally dependent upon mechanical ventilation and thus will be kept alive with the ventilator. There are a number of issues to consider with such round-the-clock noninvasive or invasive ventilation. The most important is that when the patient uses full-time ventilation the progression of ALS does not stop. Strength will continue to be lost just as before respiratory failure. With noninvasive ventilation, speech will be lost eventually, and it will be lost when invasive ventilation is started.

It is most important to understand that patients can choose to extend their lives using either noninvasive or invasive ventilation or can choose not to extend their lives (as discussed below). Which course is chosen and which type of ventilator is used should be discussed with the neurologist and pulmonologist.

More about Noninvasive Ventilation

Noninvasive ventilation is most commonly used for obstructive sleep apnea, in which case a constant stream of air is provided; the formal term is continuous positive airway pressure (CPAP). In ALS, more air pressure is required than with CPAP, and it would be taxing for the patient to exhale against the higher pressure. Accordingly, the ventilator used for ALS patients has two pressure settings. The pressure settings may be adjusted to support progressive weakness of the diaphragm. BiPAP is the brand name of a **bilevel noninvasive ventilation** device. Other relevant abbreviations are NIV (noninvasive ventilation) or NPPV (noninvasive positive pressure ventilation).

The bilevel ventilator is a small box that requires household AC current, and some ventilators of this type also have a battery for limited away-from-home use. The ventilator has a hose that connects to an interface, described above. The fit of the interface is important, as patient faces differ in shape and the interface has to fit comfortably. It may take a trial of several interfaces to find a good fit. Most noninvasive ventilators have a humidifier to make the airstream less dry.

Since breathing is compromised during sleep, the goal is to use noninvasive ventilation at least 4 hours per night, and more is better. Some patients feel that they get a better night's sleep with it. Some people use it during naps, as they feel more rested afterward. Other patients experience no change, even though the neurologist may feel that they are getting some benefit from using it.

Patients may have difficulty adjusting to using noninvasive ventilation. They feel that it is "controlling their breathing," when it is actually responding to their breathing cycles. It may make them feel "closed in" or claustrophobic. There are several suggestions for managing claustrophobia. One is for patients to use noninvasive ventilation first for brief periods during the day while awake, then use it during naps, and gradually use it for longer periods, finally using it at night. Use can be a challenge for patients with arm and hand weakness, who may not be able to take the mask off if they feel the need to. Despite best efforts, a number of patients cannot get comfortable with noninvasive ventilation, and that is all right.

For the patient using noninvasive ventilation 24 hours a day, their cough will be inadequate and they will need to rely upon a CoughAssist device to clear secretions.

What Is Diaphragm Pacing?

"Diaphragm pacing" refers to electrically activating the diaphragm more fully than the patient can typically achieve by natural breathing. The goals are to perhaps strengthen the diaphragm and to reduce atelectasis. Diaphragm pacing is used with noninvasive ventilation, mainly at night. To enable diaphragm pacing, fine wires are inserted into the underside of the diaphragm (one set in each hemidiaphragm) during a laparoscopic surgical procedure performed under general anesthesia; this surgery has a small risk of complications. The wires come out of the body just under the ribcage and are connected to an electrical stimulator, which, when activated, causes the diaphragm to contract at a rate of approximately 12 times per minute.

It is essential to understand that the electrical stimulation of the diaphragm occurs by the electrodes' activating the phrenic nerves as they enter the diaphragm. Thus the effects of diaphragm pacing are limited by the number of lower motor nerve fibers in the phrenic nerves. Some patients may have too few nerve fibers and cannot receive the device. With all patients, as ALS progresses, there will be fewer and fewer phrenic nerve fibers, and use of diaphragm pacing will become limited.

The benefits of diaphragm pacing are not clear at this time, and until more data are available its use in ALS is not encouraged.

More about Invasive Ventilation

Invasive ventilation is called invasive because the normal pathway of air from the nose or mouth to the lungs is altered. As mentioned earlier, occasionally a patient may need to be ventilated in an emergency situation, in which case an endotracheal tube can be placed without a surgical procedure. This tube can be used for up to 2 weeks before it must be replaced by a tracheal tube, because using an endotracheal tube for longer periods of time will damage the trachea. It is also uncomfortable for the patient to have a tube passing through their throat. The goal of inserting an endotracheal tube is to rapidly establish ventilation and allow time for the patient to make a decision whether to continue with tracheal ventilation or to be allowed to pass away peacefully.

Invasive ventilation provides sufficient oxygen and removes carbon dioxide. The patient does not need to make an effort to breathe and is comfortable, with no shortness of breath. Within a short amount of time on a ventilator, there is total dependence upon the ventilator, 24 hours a day. With good care, a patient can live for years using artificial ventilation.

Issues particular to invasive ventilation include that after the tracheal tube is in place, air will no longer pass over the vocal cords. If speech was not possible before the tracheostomy, it will still not be possible after. If speech was possible before, after the incision for the tracheal tube heals, a special tracheal tube can be used that allows some air to leak past and across the vocal cords, permitting speech. However, control of the vocal cords will be impaired as ALS progresses and speech may not continue to be possible. Alternative means of communication can then be used. With further time, movement will be reduced, and it may be difficult to communicate even by making yes/no gestures, including blinking the eyes.

With tracheal ventilation the patient will no longer be able to cough. A cough requires a deep breath and forceful expiration against the closed larynx. The tracheal tube effectively prevents closure of the larynx, so no pressure can be built up. Therefore secretions must be manually cleared, using a simple procedure. A caregiver places a thin tube into the airway and applies suction to clear the secretions.

It is important to consider that if a patient has been on hospice care and begins to use invasive ventilation, he or she cannot remain in hospice. Hospice care enters the picture when there are no treatments that will reverse the course of the disease, and hospice will not provide treatment in a manner that will prolong survival. Nocturnal noninvasive ventilation can be considered comfort care, but converting to invasive ventilation represents prolonging survival. It is not clear how hospice will respond when a patient who has been using noninvasive ventilation at night needs to use it 24 hours a day.

The patient on a ventilator cannot be left alone, because he or she is dependent upon the ventilator and has weak limbs from ALS. In the rare event of a problem with the ventilator or a connection, it is likely that the patient would die before the caregiver returned. Twenty-four-hour care requires caregivers to take shifts. It can be managed with family and friends or with the use of hired attendants. In our ALS clinic, we discuss these issues early on when patients and families ask about use of invasive or 24-hour noninvasive ventilation. We conclude by saying that such ventilation can be managed.

Further issues include providing for a backup supply of electricity (a generator) in case of a power failure. In emergency situations the local fire station will have electricity from a generator, and the station should be notified that there is a patient dependent on a ventilator in the area. Converters also are available for using current from an automobile. In addition, a second ventilator should be obtained in case there is an issue with the one being used.

How Do I Make the Choice for or against Full-Time Ventilation?

Whether to choose to remain on full-time ventilation (24 hours a day, 7 days a week) is perhaps the most difficult question for the patient.

It is a question of whether to let ALS follow its natural progression to death or to prolong survival with artificial means. This is a personal decision and will depend upon a number of factors. One is whether the patient has particular events that he or she wants to participate in, such as weddings or births, and following the events can be made comfortable and allowed to pass away. Another important consideration is whether a patient's family is encouraging invasive ventilation when the patient is less inclined to use it or, conversely, the patient desires invasive ventilation while the family does not feel capable of sustaining the required level of care for either practical or financial reasons. Finally, there is the patient's fear of death without invasive ventilation.

As previously discussed, sometimes the question of whether to use invasive ventilation arises under emergency circumstances when acute shortness of breath occurs, and the decision must be made quickly in the hospital. In some cases the patient cannot actively contribute to the decision to intubate or not. These are uncommon but not rare circumstances in ALS. To anticipate situations of this sort, it is important that the patient consider, and reconsider periodically, what he or she would wish with respect to invasive ventilation. These wishes should be discussed with family members and ideally written in a living will or power of attorney for medical affairs (see Chapter 16). The least comfortable situation for the patient and family is to "back into" having a tracheostomy when it was not desired. However, it is important to know that if this situation arises and the patient is started on invasive ventilation, but subsequently makes clear that he or she does not want the invasive ventilation, breathing support can be stopped and the patient can be made comfortable and allowed to pass away, as discussed at the end of this chapter.

What Does "Locked in" Mean?

Being in a **locked-in** state means that a patient can hear, feel, and understand but cannot express or communicate his or her needs or concerns: he or she is "locked in" the body and cannot get anything out. This is not a comfortable state for the patient, caregiver, family, or medical personnel. Becoming locked-in rarely happens with ALS in the United States, but if a patient has been on invasive ventilation or 24-hour noninvasive ventilation for a long time (years) and weakness has progressed, he or she may not be able to respond with gestures or use eye movements to answer questions.

What If I No Longer Want to Continue Full-Time Ventilation?

When patients with ALS choose full-time ventilation (noninvasive or invasive), it is reasonable to expect that at some time they will have accomplished their personal goals and will want to pass away comfortably. At this time, the patient can be placed on hospice care, made comfortable, and allowed to pass away peacefully (see Chapter 15). As weakness progresses while the patient is on full-time ventilation, it is important for the neurologist, pulmonologist, and family to ask if the patient is satisfied with his or her quality of life. The patient should make his or her decision about ventilation known before progressing to the stage of being locked-in and unable to express thoughts, concerns, and wishes.

Chapter 11

Communication and ALS

How Does ALS Affect Speech?

Communication through speaking is an essential human trait allowing people to share a range of thoughts from basic needs to complex issues. Normally, this occurs without effort, and each participant exchanges words easily. In ALS, two issues can arise that affect communication, and the majority of patients will experience one or both of them.

The loss of upper and lower motor neurons reduces the ability to speak clearly. This is called **dysarthria**. Initially, patients will work harder to be understood, and even with moderately severe dysarthria, patients can usually communicate basic needs, especially with familiar listeners. At some point when the dysarthria has progressed, the difficulty shifts to the listener, because the patient can no longer articulate sufficiently clearly. This leads to frustration on the part of both the speaker and listener, and the patient may give up trying to communicate. This can leave both parties stressed and angry. It is also during this stage that patients most feel the need to talk about complex issues such as end-of-life decisions. As a result, these thoughts become very difficult to communicate when dysarthria increases in severity. A speech-language pathologist can make useful suggestions about ways to facilitate communication.

The second issue occurs in patients who also have FTLD, which impairs language. As a result the patient may think of and say fewer words.

How Can Speech Be Optimized?

Factors other than dysarthria can also prevent the patient from speaking optimally. For example, fatigue reduces both clarity and endurance for longer conversations. Patients often find that expressing complex issues early in the day is more successful. For the listener, directly attending to the patient is important: television sets should be off, and conversations should ideally occur face-to-face, as this positioning optimizes concentration and the reading of lips and facial expressions. The benefit of lip-reading and seeing facial expressions can be appreciated by considering that it is more difficult to communicate over the telephone with a person with ALS. Keeping questions and answers simple will also reduce frustration for both the patient and the listener.

When dysarthria increases and speech becomes more challenging, patients may benefit from augmenting their communication or using an alternative means of communication. Many aids and devices are available that can be used as needs increase. A speech-language pathologist and occupational therapist can be helpful in identifying those that best meet the patient's needs. They range from "low-tech" aids to more complex, "high-tech" aids. Not every patient with ALS will need the full spectrum of these devices or other aids, but they can reduce frustrations. It is important to note that these alternative means are less effective when the problem is reduced word output due to FTLD. In that circumstance, asking direct yes/no questions may be more successful.

What Are Low-Tech Speech Aids?

Low-tech speech aids are simple devices that are readily available in the home or are inexpensive.

Handwriting

When speech becomes harder, writing is a natural alternative. While slower than speech, handwriting allows both simple and complex messages to be easily communicated. The patient may carry a small notebook to write messages in or use a small dry-erase "whiteboard." The latter option is beneficial when hand weakness makes it difficult to hold a pen, as a whiteboard is written on with a large-diameter marker. Occupational therapists can recommend adaptive aids to assist patients in holding or gripping a pen to maintain the ability to write. When holding a pen is not possible, writing with the finger on touch-sensitive tablets or with certain applications ("apps") on digital tablets can be used.

Alphabet Board

Patients with ALS or family members can construct simple alphabet boards with letters arranged in alphabetical or QWERTY (keyboard) order. Alphabet boards can be used to supplement speech by having the ALS patient point to the first letter of each word along with speaking the message. When using this "alphabet supplementation" method, the patient speaks at a slow rate and the listener sees the first letter of each word, which often helps to increase speech intelligibility in the setting of moderate dysarthria. The patient spells out any words that are missed. Patients with no functional speech can spell out complete messages on the alphabet board. Communication can be speeded up by including on the board frequently used words and phrases involving daily care needs.

If the patient cannot point, the listener can move his or her finger over letters or phrases on the board, and the patient indicates in some way (nods, eye-blinks) when the message element is reached. Another approach is to use a transparent alphabet board with the listener on one side and the patient on the opposite side; here the listener tracks the patient's direction of gaze to the letters that spell out words. Patients with adequate head control can also use an adapted laser pointer attached to a cap or to a pair of eyeglasses to select letters or phrases on the alphabet board.

> Lois experienced severe dysarthria early in the course of her disease. Handwriting notes to caregivers and others proved to be her most effective method of communication, and she was able to write until very near the end of her life. Lois was particularly close to her twin sister, Lorene, and enjoyed visiting her in the city, when the two of them would sit for hours with Lois writing and Lorene speaking. It was a healthy release for Lois to be able to convey her thoughts about her condition clearly to her twin, and she was fortunate to be able to communicate fluently this way.

What Are Medium-Tech Speech Aids?

Medium-tech speech aids are readily available devices that can be adapted for use in the setting of dysarthria.

Speech Amplification

For some patients with ALS, an early change in speech is softness of the voice. The patient who continues to work may need to amplify his or her speech in order to speak in the workplace. Whether at work, in the home, or elsewhere, a head-mounted microphone connected to an amplifier-speaker can reduce the effort of voice projection.

Mobile Telephones

Mobile telephones allow ALS patients with reasonable manual dexterity to type messages that can be read by the listener or sent as a text message or email. Mobile telephones with advanced operating systems (smartphones) can be set to read text or email messages aloud using synthesized speech.

Digital Tablets

The larger keyboard on a digital tablet can be used for typing in the same way as the keyboard on a mobile telephone. For both, an ever-growing variety of free and low-cost speech-generating applications are available that will convert written text into synthesized spoken text.

What Are High-Tech Speech Aids?

When a patient loses the ability to speak and can no longer use his or her hands to write, to point to an alphabet board, or to access a keyboard or touchscreen, specialized high-tech speech aids are available to help maintain communication. High-tech augmentative and alternative communication (AAC) devices include computers that allow the patient to construct messages and speak them using a speech synthesizer. Messages are created using spelling, combinations of preprogrammed, commonly used phrases, or both.

Head- and Eye-Tracking Devices

Head-tracking and **eye-gaze technologies** are used to highlight letters, words, or symbols on the computer. Head-tracking devices use an infrared sensor to track a reflective "dot" attached to the user's forehead in order to determine what item the user is looking at. Eye tracking works in a similar manner, but instead of following head movement, the device tracks the user's eye movements. A computer program combines the letters into words and then expresses them as readable (on the computer screen) or as synthesized spoken words. The messages can also be sent as emails, and the computer can also be used to surf the Web. Calibrating the patient's head or eye movements on the screen can be challenging, and periodic adjustments are needed as the patient becomes weaker. Medicare, Medicaid, and most private insurance cover these devices, but to receive coverage the patient must have an evaluation by a speech-language pathologist, who will submit a written report for prior authorization.

> For John, ALS started with hand weakness. When John's voice became slurred, he and his wife had difficulty communicating, as he could not even hold a pen to write. He and his family started using an alphabet board to aid their communication and eventually turned to an eye-gaze computer interface. It was slow going for him to pick out letters, but he was able to make his thoughts known to his family and also send emails and surf the Web.

Voice Banking

Before dysarthria becomes severe, patients may "bank" their own voices to be used on their communication devices. Voice banking involves digitally recording words and sentences read by the patient; a special computer program can then use these digital files to create a synthetic voice quite close to the speaker's natural voice. This more natural voice can be used on computer devices when the patient spells out words and sentences and the device speaks them. It is important that a patient look ahead and bank words before speech becomes slurred.

Brain-Computer Interface Communication

A **brain-computer interface** communication system records brainwaves using an electrode array on the patient's scalp and translates them into a moving dot on a computer screen that the patient controls to spell out words. While this technology is very attractive, it is in early development. It is also more difficult to use than other technologies, because for every use, electrodes must be applied to the scalp by another person and remain in intimate contact with the scalp during use. Moreover, the machine must be calibrated to the patient's brainwaves, and the patient must learn how to harness his or her thoughts to spell words.

Chapter 12

Mobility and ALS

"Mobility" is used here as the general term for the use of arms, hands, and legs to accomplish activities of daily living. With ALS, managing activities of daily living becomes a challenge in adaptation and inventiveness. The progression of weakness and the need to continually adapt and reinvent are somewhat unique to ALS, and the process is challenging and tiring for the spirit. For athletically inclined ALS patients, adaptations can be made to equipment and techniques can be altered to allow activities such as cycling, skiing, hiking, and other sports to be pursued when impairments are mild. When weakness progresses, adaptations can be made for bathing, dressing, eating, writing, and typing; mechanical aids can help compensate for greater weakness later on. Difficulty walking can be an early problem with ALS, but even if not an early problem, it will become an issue with most patients over the course of the disease. Walking difficulties increase the risk of falls and injury, and falls can be the first indication of leg difficulties leading to the diagnosis of ALS. Once walking difficulties are experienced, it is important to learn to manage safe transfers in and out of the tub or shower, in and out of bed, from the bed to a wheelchair, on and off the toilet, and so forth. Weakness and stiffness of legs (spasticity) can affect limb movements and driving. Equipment such as canes, walkers, and wheelchairs can make a large difference in safe function. Finally, adaptations to the home can have a major impact on daily function.

How Can I Pursue Athletic Activities?

The ability to continue with such activities depends upon the distribution of weakness, the type of activity and equipment used, and the inventiveness of the patient and occupational and physical therapists. As examples, cycling with some hand weakness can be managed with modifications to the position of brake levers and with the use of one lever to control both brakes. Patients can switch from riding a single bicycle to taking the stoker position on a tandem bike. Stability while hiking can be improved by using two trekking poles. Various swimming strokes can be used when the arms and legs are weak. Most university medical centers have rehabilitation clinics that can work with clinic therapists and the patient. With pursuit of athletic activities comes an overall concern for patient safety that must be addressed.

How Can I Manage Dressing?

Many clothing features can make getting dressed and undressed challenging, but adaptive aids are available that can ease the process. The occupational therapist in the clinic can help with suggestions. An alternative is changing the style of clothes one wears to types that simplify the process of dressing and undressing. The following are some ways of making dressing easier:

- A buttonhook can make the process of buttoning easier when finger dexterity is compromised.
- Replacing buttons with small circles of Velcro, with hooks on one side and loops on the other, can allow use of shirts with plackets. Snaps, as on Western-style shirts, are easier to do up and undo than are regular buttons.
- Zipper pulls can be fashioned from a loop of monofilament fishing line or a small split key ring. Alternatively, a small pair of vice grip pliers can be used to grasp the zipper tab when needed.

- Loose-fitting athletic warm-up pants with elastic waistbands are easier to put on and take off than conventional pants with buttons, belts, and zippers. For women who spend most time in a wheelchair, there are open skirts that clip around the waist.
- Shoelaces or sneaker laces can be replaced with elastic ones that are permanently tied. A shoehorn with a long handle reduces the need to bend over when stepping into shoes.

How Can I Get on and off the Toilet?

This is a many-times-a-day issue and is associated with falls. The process requires loosening and pulling clothes up or down, turning around, lowering oneself onto the toilet, and rising when finished. For support getting on and off the toilet many people use a bathroom vanity cabinet near the toilet, but cabinets are usually only on one side of the toilet and often are some distance away from the toilet. Easy-to-attach toilet seat replacements are available that have bars at the side to ease lowering and rising. Some have associated risers to make the toilet seat higher. Examples can be found on the Internet (search for "handicap bathroom aids"). An alternative is a commode that can be used in any room or placed over the toilet. If these stationary aids are not sufficient because of leg weakness, power-operated lift seats can be placed over the toilet, allowing the patient to be lowered and raised without using his or her own effort. The drawback is that these are more expensive than other options.

How Can I Get in and out of the Shower and Tub?

Showers

Showers traditionally have a ridge to step over. Grab handles can be positioned to aid the patient in stepping into and out of the shower.

If this becomes a challenge, consideration should be given to renovating the shower to eliminate the ridge. Generally, one stands during a shower, which is difficult for many patients. If the shower does not have a built-in bench, a shower chair can be used. To reduce body movements in the shower, one can replace the fixed shower water nozzle with a wand nozzle that is easily used to rinse all parts of the body. Body movements needed when drying with a towel can challenge a patient's balance, and drying by putting on an absorbent terry cloth robe may be safer.

When traveling, one may find that showers in public accommodations do not have grab handles. Taking along a portable grab handle that can be easily affixed to the shower wall with suction cups can add an element of safety.

Bathtubs

Bathtubs pose the challenges of getting over the side of the tub, lowering oneself to a lying position, and then moving from a lying to a standing position. Handles that can be clamped onto the tub to help are available for purchase. Some companies can cut a door in a tub, or a replacement walk-in tub can be installed with remodeling of the bathroom. Examples are available on the Internet (search for "walk-in tubs").

How Do I Manage Personal Hygiene?

Everyone has a sense of personal space, and hygiene associated with bowel movements is an important example. When hands become too weak to manage this process, use of a special bidet permits personal control over hygiene. The original bidet is a separate basin the size and position of a toilet, and the user cleans himself or herself by washing with water, soap, and a washcloth. However, a type of bidet is available from major toilet manufacturers in the form of a replacement toilet seat. The bidet toilet seat has the ability to spritz warm water onto the patient's bottom (perineal area), followed by warm air for drying, all at the press of a button. Installation is straightforward but requires connecting the waterline to the toilet's tank and connecting to AC power for the spritzer pump and to warm the water. Toilet seat bidets can be found on the Internet (search for "bidet toilet seats").

How Do I Manage Brushing My Teeth with Weak Hands?

Dental hygiene is important, and when hand and arm weakness prevents easy use of a conventional toothbrush, an electric toothbrush can be used. An electric toothbrush has several advantages over a manual one: the handle is larger and easier to hold; a built-in timer assures a full 2 minutes of brushing; and if a caregiver has to manipulate the toothbrush, using an electric toothbrush accomplishes a more thorough brushing than if the caregiver has to make all of the movements.

How Can I Turn Over in Bed?

As legs become weak or stiff, it can become difficult to turn over in bed. Feet frequently get caught up in the sheets and blankets during the turning maneuver. Further, legs and buttocks may not slide easily over the sheets when the patient is getting into and out of bed and during turning. Arm weakness can complicate the process. Several adjustments can be made:

- Construction of a "blanket tent" at the foot of the bed elevates the sheets and blankets off the patient's feet. A cardboard box with a large opening cut in one of the long sides can be used, with the patient's feet in the box and the sheets and blankets over the box. A metal frame can also be purchased.

- Use of satin pajamas and sheets can reduce friction, compared with regular cotton pajamas and cotton sheets, when the patient is sliding into or out of bed and during turning maneuvers.
- Use of a frame with a bar (trapeze) over the bed can provide a handhold for the patient when turning.
- A variety of bedrails are available that can be easily attached to a bed and used as handholds.
- Vertical poles that can be positioned near the bed and secured between the floor and ceiling by expanding their length can be used as handholds.

How Can I Support My Head and Back?

Some patients with ALS have weakness of the neck extensor muscles, which hold up the head, causing the patient's neck to become sore when standing and walking. The human head is heavy, weighing about 12 pounds, and when neck muscles weaken, the head can drop. This can be managed early on by using a soft foam collar when walking or when in a vehicle to reduce movements from acceleration and stopping and from irregularities in the road. When weakness becomes marked, firm collars can be worn. However, the firmer the collar, the harder it is to move the jaw to produce speech, which may already have become difficult to understand by this time. The most practical solution is rotating among different styles of collar.

Similarly, some patients experience weakness of the thoracic spine and tend to bend over when walking. When muscles surrounding the spine become weak, patients cannot stand erect (straight). Chest or thoracic braces can be tried to compensate for these difficulties, but the tighter they are, the more confining they feel. The best option is to use a walker, with arm muscles providing some of the support that spine muscles cannot.

Why Do I Feel Unsteady and Fall?

In ALS, walking is affected by two factors: one is lower motor neuron loss resulting in weakness of muscles needed for walking, and the other is upper motor neuron loss leading to gait spasticity. The two frequently occur together. Walking on two feet is a major feat of balance. Watching a toddler learn to walk shows how much leg muscles work to keep the center of gravity under the body. Although toddlers easily learn to walk, run, hop, skip, and jump, the smoothness of these activities is dependent upon getting nerve signals from balance centers in the brain down to muscles before gravity takes over. In ALS, the balance centers are working well, but the loss of upper motor neurons prevents the commands from traveling down the spinal cord and out to muscles before normal degrees of being off balance become irreversible. Further, muscles that are weak because of the loss of lower motor neurons cannot move the body back in place with sufficient force.

Lower motor neuron loss in the legs in ALS most commonly causes footdrop, usually initially on one side. Footdrop results when weakness of the muscles about the shin causes an inability to pick up the toes as the leg swings through. This leads to "catching one's toe" and stumbling. Occasionally, a person with undiagnosed ALS may not appreciate this weakness, fall, and break a bone, and discover, when he or she starts to walk again after the cast or splint is removed, that muscle weakness is causing difficulty bending the foot at the ankle, despite physical therapy. In this situation, weakness due to ALS caused the fall, but the underlying disease became clear only with the progression of weakness over time.

Thigh muscles can become weak in ALS, and patients then have difficulty rising from low seats (chairs, couches, toilet seats) without pushing off with their arms from the armrests. They may be very unsteady during the transition from sitting to standing to starting to walk. Thigh muscle weakness can also cause a leg to unexpectedly give out at the knee, resulting in a fall.

Upper motor neuron loss causes muscles not to contract and relax in a smooth manner, resulting in stiffness of gait. Muscles normally work in opposite pairs: one set flexes and the other set extends. When flexor muscles are activated, extensor muscles are quiet, and vice versa. With spasticity, however, when flexor muscles are activated, extensor muscles remain partially active, and one set of muscles fights against the other, causing the patient's walking to resemble that of Frankenstein's monster. When the patient tries to regain balance, there is a battle of muscles between flexors and extensors, and balance is impaired.

Spasticity can also cause a toe to catch and thereby lead to a stumble. However, spasticity can be less obvious: the patient simply feels "unbalanced" and may fall suddenly when leaning forward, bending down, or turning. This occurs because with any leaning, a person is mildly off balance. As described above, with ALS the commands from the balance center to muscles are slow and do not occur in time to correct being off balance. Patients frequently report they "fall hard," with no ability to take a quick step to regain their center of gravity.

An interesting phenomenon due to spasticity is greater stiffness with the first steps as compared with later steps after a patient has been sitting for a long time and begins walking. Thus falls are more common with the first few steps. The explanation for this is not clear, but it is likely that nerve activity related to muscles working and joints moving (also called **proprioceptive** activity) increases after a few steps and helps reduce the effect of muscles fighting against each other.

For all types of walking difficulties, patients with ALS must concentrate on how they are walking and be vigilant about where they are walking. Turns must be slow and controlled: make the turn and then start walking again. Concentration is reduced when one is in a hurry, distracted by carrying something, or tired. Patients should be very careful when leaning forward or stooping down. In fact, many patients should not lean down to pick things up! Remembering to take this degree of care with walking can be difficult, because after learning to walk as toddlers, we get up, walk, turn, and bend without thought.

The fatigue of walking to and from the car in a parking lot can be reduced by parking in a handicapped space. The ALS clinic can provide a form to obtain a handicapped license plate or placard.

What Can Be Done to Aid Walking?

A number of simple aids are available to make walking easier. It is common that a patient will start with one walking aid, will need another aid with the progression of weakness over time, and eventually will require a wheelchair.

Ankle-Foot Orthosis

With a mild footdrop, being aware of the difficulty may be sufficient for safe walking. This means that one must watch how and where one walks. As the footdrop progresses, a brace across the ankle that holds the foot at a right angle to the leg can help. This brace is called an **ankle-foot orthosis (AFO)**. There are different models of AFOs, and the physical therapist works with an orthotist to determine which type would be most effective. To be effective, the AFO must be worn all the time, as patients often report falls around the house when they are not wearing it.

Cane or Walking Stick

A cane or walking stick can help provide stability and reduce the feeling of being off balance. Canes can be simple or complex with four short feet (quad cane) and should be used on the patient's strong side. A simple cane is best with ALS because it is light in weight and easier to maneuver if the patient's hand or arm is weak. A trekking pole used as a walking stick has two advantages over a cane. If the patient slips his or her hand up through the strap (as in holding a ski pole), the hand does not have to grip the handle, as a downward movement of the hand at the beginning of a fall will pull the hand into the handle and support the arm. The other advantage is that by leaning on the end of the pole, the patient can use the pole as a third leg (forming a tripod with patient's two legs) to rest.

Walker

With progression of leg weakness and spasticity, a walker can provide more stability. There are two- and four-wheeled walkers. Two-wheeled walkers have two small-diameter wheels at the front and two rear supports (usually with tennis balls attached to them) that must be slid along the ground. Four-wheeled walkers have four larger wheels (which can more easily roll over bumps and cracks) and can be pushed easily, and it is uncommon for patients to report that such walkers get away from them. It is helpful for a walker to have a seat to rest on and a basket to carry items in. Four-wheeled walkers have two lever-operated handbrakes that can be locked and are used when the patient leans on the walker while turning or to sit down or stand up. Both types of walkers can be collapsed for ease of transportation. In our ALS clinic we recommend four-wheeled walkers.

Lift Chairs

To help patients for whom rising from a chair is difficult, easy chairs are available with electric lift features that partially elevate patients when they want to stand. These patients can also use portable cushions when visiting homes with low chairs.

Medications for Spasticity

Chapter 13 discusses medications that can aid mobility by reducing spasticity due to upper motor neuron loss.

What If I Fall and Cannot Get Up (Medical Alert Signaling Systems)?

When walking is impaired, falls occur. If the patient cannot get up on his or her own and no one is at home to help, the patient may be left lying there, frightened and in pain from an injury. Commercially available signaling systems that connect to a telephone allow the patient to press a button to call preprogrammed telephone numbers to summon help. In our ALS clinic we urge patients to get such a system to remove anxiety about leaving the patient at home alone. Many companies offering such systems can be found on the Internet (search for "medical alert systems").

What about Wheelchairs?

A wheelchair can be thought of as a tool, one that allows the patient to move farther, faster, and with less fatigue. There are two types of wheelchairs, manual and power. Each has advantages, and many patients benefit from having both.

Manual Wheelchairs

Manual wheelchairs have two large wheels toward the back and two small wheels in the front. They should be of the lightweight variety, about 20 pounds, and be collapsible. This means that they will be portable and can be kept in the back of a vehicle and used whenever the opportunity arises to do something some distance away from the vehicle. It is not expected that the patient will propel the wheelchair; rather, a caregiver will push it.

There is also a transfer wheelchair, which has four small wheels and is designed to be used inside and on smooth floors. It can be used only for limited travel outside, as the small wheels do not roll easily over sidewalk cracks and bumps.

Power Wheelchairs

Power wheelchairs have motors and a controller, usually a joystick, that the patient operates to accelerate, slow down, and steer. Patients who use power wheelchairs usually have considerable leg weakness and frequently spend more time during the day in the power wheelchair than in any other chair. Power wheelchairs should be equipped with tilt and recline features to change the patient's position and relieve pressure on the buttocks, back, and shoulders.

How Do I Get a Power Wheelchair in and out of the House and Car?

A ramp is needed to use a wheelchair outside the house. The slope of the ramp is important to consider, as are turns in the ramp if needed. An informative website that discusses dimensions and features for ramps is assistutah.org.

Power wheelchairs are heavy, between 250 and 350 pounds, and a suitable vehicle is necessary to transport the wheelchair when one is out and about. Such vehicles are usually modified, wheelchair-accessible vans. Certain companies can modify the height of a van (whether already owned or newly purchased) to accommodate a person in a wheelchair. Vans can include ramps that allow patients to transport themselves into the van, after which the wheelchair is strapped down.

If the resources for a suitable vehicle are unavailable, having both types of wheelchairs is usually necessary: a power chair for mobility within the house and in the neighborhood, and a manual chair in the family vehicle for use farther away from the home.

Does Insurance Pay for a Wheelchair?

The cost of a manual wheelchair is $2,000 to $2,500, while that of a power wheelchair is $25,000 to $30,000. Insurance often covers the cost of one wheelchair. Therefore it is most cost-effective for the patient to purchase the manual wheelchair with personal funds and the power wheelchair through the insurance. Some ALS clinics have a loan closet and can provide either type of wheelchair. If the ALS patient is a military veteran and has registered with a veterans medical center, he or she may be provided with a power wheelchair, ramps, and possibly a van.

How Do I Order a Wheelchair?

Manual and power wheelchairs must be properly fitted to the patient. The fitting is done by a physical therapist with experience in this area and supported by the wheelchair vendor. Both types of wheelchairs must have the correct height, width, length to foot supports, and position of arm supports. The power drive for power wheelchairs can be configured to drive the front wheels, middle wheels, or rear wheels, with differences in turning radius and other features that affect handling. Thus it is essential that selection and fit be conducted in the patient's home.

Because power wheelchairs are very expensive, insurance companies (including Medicare) require a formal evaluation of need by a physician within a short period of time before placing the order. After insurance grants preapproval, it can take 6 to 12 weeks to receive the wheelchair. During this period, ALS will progress, so patients are encouraged to start the process early.

What about a Scooter?

The question frequently arises as to whether a scooter may be used in place of a power wheelchair. While an attractive option when walking is only mildly impaired, a scooter does not offer sufficient support when legs become weaker, and it requires good arm and hand strength to steer and manipulate the speed lever. The legs and arms of most patients with ALS will gradually become weaker and they will not be able to control a scooter; thus it is not a good choice for the long term.

Scooter companies advertise that insurance will cover the cost of a scooter. However, the scooter counts as "power mobility," and if insurance is used to obtain it, insurance will likely not cover the cost of a proper power wheelchair when the need arises.

Why Are Patients Reluctant to Use Mobility Aids?

It is not uncommon that patients are reluctant to use a cane or walking stick, an AFO, a walker, or a wheelchair. Many times they feel it is "not necessary" and say they will take "more care walking." In fact, with progression of ALS some patients fall less frequently despite having greater difficulty walking, because they have more experience with what they cannot do. However, other patients continue to fall and become reluctant to move around outside because of the risks of a fall due to fatigue from walking. One can appreciate that some patients find use of a walking aid discomfiting because it is visible to everyone and signals that the patient has an infirmity. Significantly, the need for an aid also means that ALS is progressing, something patients may be reluctant to accept. These are valid concerns and feelings: that is why walking aids are presented as tools to be used, and it is hoped that patients view them as such.

It is also possible for elements of FTLD to contribute to reluctance in accepting walking aids. Patients with ALS with elements of dementia can have difficulty making the decision to use and accept aids and may be caught up in maintaining their old patterns. The best approach is steady encouragement and explanation of the benefits of their use.

How Can I Transfer Safely?

Transfers need to be done many times daily. A safe transfer can be defined as one that does not hurt or injure the patient or any person helping the patient. Most patients figure out how to transfer by themselves as they become weaker. However, a time comes when they need help. A simple hand will suffice for a while, but later more help is needed. As ALS patients weaken, they offer less and less help during transfers, and the caregiver approaches carrying all of the patient's weight ("dead weight"). There are positioning techniques for both the caregiver and patients that can reduce the potential for injuries. Instruction from a physical or occupational therapist is essential for manual transfers. The therapist should not only demonstrate transfers but also watch while the patient and caregiver carry them out. Given the progression of ALS, transfers should be reviewed with the physical and occupational therapist at every clinic visit.

As weakness progresses further, the caregiver may not be able to manage transfers. About half the time, the patient is larger and heavier than the caregiver. Sometimes other family members or friends can help when manual transfers become challenging, but they may not be available when an urgent need to be transferred arises. Under these circumstances a lift is essential. Training for use of a lift should be done in the home so the therapist can see the home environment.

What Is a Lift?

A lift is a device that can pick up the patient mechanically and move him or her from one site to another. The lifting mechanism can be manual (hydraulic system with a pump handle) or electric (electric motor). Further, the lift can rest on the floor (floor lift) or be bolted to the ceiling (ceiling lift). For all types of lifts, the patient is in a sling. Each type has advantages and disadvantages.

Floor Lifts

Floor lifts have two legs with small wheels that extend forward, but the legs make it difficult to maneuver in tight spaces and it is difficult to move the lift with the patient suspended. To minimize these problems, the lift can be positioned so that the patient is lifted up and down and moved over a short distance (from bed into a wheelchair, from a wheelchair onto and off the toilet).

Ceiling Lifts

Ceiling lifts require tracks bolted to the ceiling (usually directly into joists). Installation is relatively straightforward and does not require major structural work. The tracks are short and positioned in specific locations. Common sites are over the bed, over the toilet, and in the living room.

What about Changes and Renovations to the Home?

Homes come in many sizes and configurations. As ALS progresses, changes to the home can make a big difference to a patient's safe mobility. Steps or stairs and bathrooms are major challenges. Most homes have front or back steps, and railings are important when walking and balance become a problem. When a patient is using a wheelchair, ramps are necessary to get in and out of the house. Stairs between floors of a house usually have 13 steps, and this number can be daunting if the patient is going up and down multiple times a day. Railings on at least one side are essential. Electrical devices can be fixed to straight staircases that will lift the patient up and down and do not require renovation; these are called stair glides or stair lifts. For homes with a split-level design, a railing for the few steps is important. If the bedroom is on an upper floor, it may be beneficial to convert a room on the ground floor to a bedroom. Other renovations include ceiling lifts, discussed above. Doorways may benefit from widening to allow easy passage of a wheelchair.

Some bathrooms have no shower or tub (for example, a ground floor bathroom intended for guests), only a tub, or only a shower with a step-over lip. Under these circumstances, renovation of the bathroom can make a major difference to the patient, and one that will be appreciated several times a day. Specifications for accessible bathrooms can be found on at the website assistutah.org.

Renovations are costly and take time, and it is suggested that these be considered early on, when the need is first predicted, so that the patient can benefit from them for the longest amount of time. If the ALS patient is a military veteran and has registered with a veterans medical center, it may offer financial help for renovations.

Can I Still Drive?

The issue of driving is important for both the patient with ALS and the people who share the road with the patient. Driving can be impaired in ALS for three reasons: weakness of legs and arms from lower motor neuron loss, inability to move the feet quickly from one pedal to another due to spasticity from upper motor neuron loss, and difficulty with judgment from FTLD.

Everyone (patient, family, and providers) has a responsibility for safe driving. If there is any doubt, the patient should not drive! This can be difficult in our society, which is based on automobile transportation. However, an accident is defined as an unplanned event that could have been prevented had circumstances leading up to the accident been recognized. For ALS the three issues discussed above are circumstances that should be recognized before an accident can occur. Thus a patient's comment that "I only drive in the neighborhood" or "I only drive during the day" is not a compelling reason to allow the patient to drive.

Some patients are reluctant to give up driving. The approach our ALS clinic takes is to ask the patient's family members if they think that the patient is safe to drive. If the answer is equivocal we recommend that the patient have a formal driving evaluation; however, if the patient passes the evaluation, it is essential to appreciate that the patient's functional ability will continue to decrease over time and that repeated evaluations will be necessary.

Managing ALS Symptoms

ALS is a simple disease in that it affects only a few types of nerve cells and does not affect organs of the body. However, symptoms or problems can occur indirectly or secondarily from weakness. It is important to appreciate that not every patient with ALS will experience all symptoms, and those listed in this chapter cover a full spectrum. Most symptoms due to ALS can be treated or managed, but because ALS is a rare disease there may have been no formal treatment trials of medications to help guide choices. All neurologists or clinics have their own lists of preferred medications, and sometimes for a given patient a number of medications and doses must be tried. The treatments described in the tables in this chapter (with brand names for medications shown in parentheses after generic names) are options to investigate with the neurologist and other providers.

How Can I Manage My Saliva?

ALS does not cause excess production of saliva. Saliva comes from three paired salivary glands, and the glands are activated by nerve impulses in the autonomic nervous system. Normally, 1 to 2 quarts of saliva are produced a day, and we swallow frequently to keep up with this production, even sometimes in the middle of a long sentence. Excess saliva in ALS results when swallowing difficulties cause saliva to not be cleared and to pool in the mouth.

Oral suction can be used in these circumstances but can be cumbersome. A number of medications reduce nerve impulses to the salivary glands. While there is no harm from taking too much of such a medication, patients may be just as bothered by a dry mouth as a wet mouth. Accordingly, the patient must decide what the correct dose is. If medications are not successful, another approach is to block the effect of nerve impulses reaching the glands by injecting the glands with botulinum toxin. In severe cases that do not respond to medications or botulinum toxin, varying doses of radiation to the glands can be given so that they do not produce as much saliva.

Medications for treating excess saliva and their doses are listed in Table 13–1, but the following is a brief list of these medications and what to expect when taking them:

- Amitriptyline: Blocks the action of nerves that activate salivary glands. Common side effects include dry mouth and constipation.
- Glycopyrrolate: Blocks the action of nerves that activate salivary glands. Common side effects include dry mouth and constipation.
- Scopolamine patch: Scopolamine is absorbed across the skin. While it is traditionally used to prevent motion sickness, a side effect is to block the action of nerves that activate salivary glands.
- Atropine: Drops labeled for eye use can be placed under the tongue (sublingually) for prompt reduction of saliva production by blocking the action of nerves that activate salivary glands. The response is rapid, and the number of drops can be adjusted to the desired effect. There may be a bitter taste.
- Botulinum toxin: Blocks nerve transmission to the salivary glands and can be injected into the glands. Toxin type A or B is injected with a fine needle into the parotid and

TABLE 13-1 Medications Used to Treat Excess Saliva (Sialorrhea)

Medication	How Supplied	Uses	Preparation	Crushable	Dosage	Frequency	Side Effects
Amitriptyline (Elavil)	Prescription	Pseudobulbar affect Saliva control Sleep aid	Tablet	Yes	25 to 50 mg	At night	Anticholinergic
Atropine	Prescription	Saliva control	Drops	No	1 to 2 drops	As needed	Anticholinergic
Botulinum toxin, type A or B	Prescription	Saliva control	Injection	No	100 to 5,000 units	Every 2 to 3 months	
Glycopyrrolate (Robinul)	Prescription	Saliva control	Tablet, solution	Yes	1 to 20 mg	1 to 2 times daily	
Scopolapmine (Transderm Scop)	Prescription	Saliva control	Transdermal patch	No	1.5 mg	1 every 3 to 4 days	Anticholinergic

submandibular salivary glands. The effect lasts several
months, and the treatment needs to be renewed periodically.
- Radiation therapy to the salivary glands: X-ray or electron
beam radiation directed to the parotid salivary glands reduces
saliva production. The radiation damages the glands and thus
is permanent. Since teeth need a certain amount of saliva
to remain healthy, radiation treatment is usually used only
when all other means have failed and saliva remains a major
challenge. To prevent the patient from receiving too much
radiation, it is usually given in small doses, with periods to
observe the effect before additional doses are administered.

How Can I Manage Thick Phlegm?

Thick phlegm likely results when the water component of excess saliva
evaporates, leaving behind proteins that are part of saliva. The protein then accumulates and becomes thick. Adequate hydration keeps
the saliva watery and easier to swallow. Suction can be used to clear
phlegm, but frequently the phlegm is too far back to be reached by the
suction probe. Mucolytic agents can be used to address the problem
of thick phlegm; medications and doses are listed in Table 13–2:

- Guaifenesin: Helps reduce the viscosity (stickiness) of secretions.
- N-acetyl cysteine: Helps reduce the viscosity (stickiness) of
secretions.

What Can I Do about Muscle Cramps?

Occasional muscle cramps are common in everyone, usually in the
lower legs and at night, but cramps occur more frequently with
ALS. They may occur during everyday activities—for example, in
arm and hand muscles during movements related to dressing or

TABLE 13-2 Medications Used to Treat Excess and Thick Phlegm

Medication	How Supplied	Uses	Preparation	Crushable	Dosage	Frequency	Side Effects
Guaifenesin (Mucinex)	Over the counter	Thick secretions	Tablet, solution	No	200 to 400 mg	As needed	Anticholinergic
N-acetyl cysteine	Over the counter	Thick secretions Pain	Capsule, tablet, solution	No	600 mg	2 times daily	

in abdominal muscles when the patient is bending to tie his or her shoes. The cause is not known but is felt to be either changes in degenerating lower motor neurons or changes in muscles due to loss of lower motor neurons. Cramps are not caused by too little fluids or not enough salt (potassium) in the diet.

Treatment can be challenging. The best medication is quinine sulfate, but this medication is hard to obtain because of US Food and Drug Administration (FDA) concerns about its safety, although it is likely safe in doses used for cramps. Note that the amount of quinine in tonic water is small, and although a patient would have to drink quarts of tonic water to get any relief, it might be worth trying. A number of medications are used to treat cramps, but mexiletine is the drug of choice, having recently been found in a formal trial to be effective in reducing the frequency of cramps associated with ALS. A nonpharmaceutical approach that can be helpful if posterior leg muscles (hamstring and calf muscles) are the muscles that most commonly cramp is to stretch these muscles before bed. The following medications and their doses are listed in Table 13–3:

- Mexiletine: An old drug also used to treat cardiac rhythm abnormalities.
- Baclofen: Mechanism of action for cramps not known. Dosages greater than two tablets three times a day are rarely more effective. Side effects include sleepiness and reduced strength (not due to ALS progression) that reverse when the dose is reduced or stopped.
- Gabapentin: Mechanism of action for cramps not known.

How Can I Stop Muscle Twitches (Fasciculations)?

Fasciculations are small, brief twitches in muscle, visible or felt. They are universal in ALS and are not harmful, but can be annoying for some

TABLE 13-3 Medications Used to Treat Muscle Cramps

Medication	How Supplied	Uses	Preparation	Crushable	Dosage	Frequency	Side Effects
Mexiletine	Prescription	Muscle cramps	Capsule	Yes	150 mg	2 times daily	
Baclofen (Lioresal)	Prescription	Spasticity Cramps Fasciculations	Tablet	Yes	5 to 20 mg	3 times daily	Sedation, weakness
Gabapentin (Neurontin)	Prescription	Muscle cramps Fasciculations	Capsule, tablet, solution	Yes	300 to 900 mg	3 times daily	

patients. Fasciculations are thought to be due to degeneration of lower or upper motor neurons or both. Since fasciculations are present in many muscles at the time of diagnosis when looked for during the needle EMG study, fasciculations newly recognized by the patient should not be of concern. Unfortunately, no reliably effective medications are available to treat fasciculations, but the following medications are sometimes tried; they are listed with their doses in Table 13–4:

- Baclofen: Mechanism of action for fasciculations not known. Dosages greater than two tablets three times a day are rarely more effective. Side effects include sleepiness and reduced strength (not due to ALS progression) that reverse when the dose is reduced or stopped.
- Gabapentin: Mechanism of action for fasciculations not known.

How Can I Reduce Leg Stiffness?

Leg stiffness in ALS is due to spasticity from loss of upper motor neurons. Some ALS patients who have marked upper motor neuron loss and spasticity sometimes experience involuntary extension of their legs when they are sitting and being transferred. This is called an **extensor spasm**. Extensor spasm may actually be helpful during transfer, as the stiff legs act as a support, though in some situations stiff legs can be a hindrance.

The most important recommendation for the management of spasticity is for the patient to take care when walking, trying not to walk or turn fast. Antispasticity drugs are available and, if taken, should be started at a low dose and increased until either the maximum dose is reached or a side effect of sleepiness occurs. These medications and their doses are listed in Table 13–5:

- Baclofen: Works in the central nervous system (spinal cord) to reduce excitation of lower motor nerves. Dosages greater than

TABLE 13-4 Medications Used to Treat Muscle Twitches (Fasciculations)

Medication	How Supplied	Uses	Preparation	Crushable	Dosage	Frequency	Side Effects
Baclofen (Lioresal)	Prescription	Spasticity Cramps Fasciculations	Tablet	Yes	5 to 20 mg	3 times daily	Sedation, weakness
Gabapentin (Neurontin)	Prescription	Muscle cramps Fasciculations	Capsule, tablet, solution	Yes	300 to 900 mg	3 times daily	

TABLE 13-5 Medications Used to Treat Leg Stiffness (Spasticity)

Medication	How Supplied	Uses	Preparation	Crushable	Dosage	Frequency	Side Effects
Baclofen (Lioresal)	Prescription	Spasticity Cramps Fasciculations	Tablet	Yes	5 to 20 mg	3 times daily	Sedation, weakness
Tizanidine (Zanaflex)	Prescription	Spasticity	Tablet	Yes	4 mg	3 times daily	Sedation

two tablets three times a day are rarely more effective. Side effects include sleepiness and reduced strength (not due to ALS progression) that reverse when the dose is reduced or stopped.

- Tizanidine: Works in the central nervous system (spinal cord) to reduce excitation of lower motor nerves. Dosages greater than one tablet three times a day are rarely more effective. Side effects include sleepiness and reduced strength (not due to ALS progression) that reverse when the dose is reduced or stopped.

When spasticity is severe, another approach is placement of a baclofen pump under the skin in the lower abdomen. The pump infuses (injects) a metered amount of baclofen through a catheter (thin tube) into the spinal fluid that surrounds the spinal cord where it is needed. In this way, high doses circulating in the blood that cause side effects can be avoided. A test dose is given during a lumbar puncture (spinal tap) to determine whether a baclofen pump would be effective. The test times the patient walking a set distance before and after injection of baclofen into the spinal fluid to determine the effectiveness of the dose. If the test dose is effective, the catheter and pump are placed by a neurosurgeon.

How Can I Manage Sudden Urges to Urinate?

There is normally time to make one's way to the bathroom comfortably when the bladder feels full. However, as discussed in Chapter 6, with ALS there can be sudden, overwhelming urgency, and patients may not make it to the bathroom without wetting themselves. The cause of urinary urgency in ALS is not known, but it is likely related to a lack of upper motor neuron control of bladder inhibition. True incontinence, where individuals wet themselves without the urge to urinate, is very rare in ALS.

It is important that a patient not limit fluid intake to reduce the frequency of going to the bathroom, because this may cause dehydration and other problems. To prevent wetting oneself, the patient should keep a regular schedule of going to the bathroom and can use a urinal or one of the following types of catheters:

- Men can use an external (condom) catheter that covers the penis like a condom and is connected to a tube that drains into a bag. It is changed daily.
- Men and women can use an indwelling bladder catheter that enters the bladder and drains into a bag. It must be changed every 3 to 4 weeks by a nurse and can increase the chance of bladder infections.
- Men and women can use a suprapubic bladder catheter that is placed in the bladder, passes through the skin, comes out just above the pubic bone, and drains into a bag. It is placed during an operative procedure and can increase the chance of bladder infections.

The following medications used to treat urinary urgency are listed with their doses in Table 13–6:

- Oxybutynin: Blocks certain neurotransmitter receptors in the bladder. It is available in different formulations. It should not be used if the patient has glaucoma. Common side effects include dry mouth and constipation.
- Tolterodine: Blocks certain neurotransmitter receptors in the bladder. Common side effects include dry mouth and constipation.

How Do I Manage Constipation?

Constipation appears to be more common as people age, but a large number of patients with ALS report constipation that is new since the diagnosis. Constipation in the setting of ALS likely

TABLE 13–6 Medications Used to Treat Urinary (Bladder) Urgency

Medication	How Supplied	Uses	Preparation	Crushable	Dosage	Frequency	Side Effects
Oxybutynin (Ditropan)	Prescription	Urinary urgency	Tablet IR	Yes	5 mg	1 to 3 times daily	Anticholinergic
Oxybutynin (Oxytrol)	Over the counter	Urinary urgency	Tablet XL	No	5 mg	1 daily	
			Transdermal patch	No	3.9 mg	1 every 3 to 4 days	
Tolterodine (Detrol)	Prescription	Urinary urgency	Tablet	Yes	2 mg	2 times daily	
			Capsule	No	2 mg	2 times daily	

has several causes, including an altered daily bathroom schedule (some people have regular bowel movements, and difficulty getting to the bathroom may alter the schedule) and relative physical inactivity (forced change to a sedentary lifestyle). A patient should not reduce fluid intake in an effort to go to the bathroom less frequently.

The gastrocolic reflex, which everyone has, is reflex activity in the distal colon (rectum) within approximately 15 minutes of eating that promotes defecation. It can be reinforced by the patient's sitting on the toilet for 15 minutes daily after breakfast to help establish a bowel schedule.

Dietary modifications that can help with bowel movements and over-the-counter medications that can promote regularity are listed below:

- Fluids: about eight 8-ounce glasses of water daily
- Fiber such as dietary bran: 20 to 35 grams daily
- Bulk-forming laxatives such as psyllium: 30 grams daily
- Osmotic agents such as polyethylene glycol (brand name Miralax): 17 grams diluted in 8 ounces of fluid daily
- Stimulant laxatives such as bisacodyl or senna: 15 mg daily

What Are Anticholinergic Side Effects of Medications?

A number of medications used to treat symptoms associated with ALS interfere with the function of the neurotransmitter acetylcholine and thereby block nerve impulses in the autonomic nervous system. The result is to slow or stop secretion of saliva, slow bowel movements, and reduce bladder contractions. Side effects include dry mouth, constipation, drowsiness, difficulty urinating, and, rarely, hallucinations. Medications with these anticholinergic side effects include amitriptyline, glycopyrrolate, and oxybutynin, discussed above. The side effects increase with dosage, but in ALS the doses of these drugs are generally low and thus the side effects are generally mild. Some side effects are actually the reason the medication is given. Amitriptyline, for example, can help reduce saliva. The most common anticholinergic side effect is constipation; if there is a sufficiently positive effect of the drug then constipation can be managed to continue taking the drug.

How Do I Manage Pain?

The loss of upper and lower motor neurons in ALS does not cause pain; however, a large number of patients report a variety of painful conditions. Pain in ALS is frequently attributed to relative immobility due to weakness and the inability to change position. People without weakness are constantly changing position and spend a relatively short time in a single position. Patients with ALS spend many hours sitting and may not be able to shift position easily. The same situation occurs during sleep: people without weakness change position many times during the night, but patients with ALS may be unable to make these changes. Weakness can also limit the ability to stretch muscles and ligaments, and joints can become tight and painful, most commonly at the shoulder (frozen shoulder). Sometimes a shoulder joint or other region of the body can be injured during a transfer.

   Pain in ALS can be managed in several ways. One is by providing assistance to the patient to change position on a regular basis. This requires time from the caregiver. Another is regular application of a stretching program for tight joints (particularly the shoulder) under the guidance of a physical therapist. This also requires caregiver time. Power wheelchairs should give patients the ability to adjust the tilt of the back of the chair and to recline. Finally, pain-relieving medications should be offered. Pain-relieving medications range from mild to narcotic analgesics and should be considered in

TABLE 13-7 Medications Used to Treat Pain

Medication	How Supplied	Uses	Preparation	Crushable	Dosage	Frequency	Side Effects
Gabapentin (Neurontin)	Prescription	Muscle cramps Fasciculations	Capsule, tablet, solution	Yes	300 to 900 mg	3 times daily	
Hydrocodone/ acetaminophen (Lortab)	Prescription	Pain	Tablet, solution	No	5 to 10 mg	2 to 4 times daily	Sedation, constipation. Limit acetaminophen to 3,000 mg per day
Ibuprofen (Advil, Motrin)	Over the counter	Pain	Tablet, solution	Yes	200 to 800 mg	3 times daily	
Lorazepam (Ativan)	Prescription	Anxiety Pain	Tablet	Yes	1 to 2 mg	As needed	Sedation
Meloxicam (Mobic)	Prescription	Pain	Tablet	Yes	7.5 to 15 mg	Daily	
Morphine sulfate	Prescription	Pain	Tablet, solution	Yes	10 to 30 mg	As needed	Sedation, constipation
N-acetyl cysteine	Over the counter	Thick secretions Pain	Capsule, tablet, solution	No	600 mg	2 times daily	
Naproxen sodium (Aleve)	Over the counter	Pain	Tablet	Yes	220 to 550 mg	2 times daily	
Dextromethorphan/ quinidine (Nuedexta)	Prescription	Pseudobulbar affect Pain	Capsule	No	20/10 mg	2 times daily	
Tramadol (Ultram)	Prescription	Pain	Tablet	No	50 mg	3 to 4 times daily	Sedation, constipation

an ascending order of potency until relief is achieved. The following medications and their doses are listed in Table 13–7:

- Nonsteroidal anti-inflammatory drugs (NSAIDs): ibuprofen, naproxen sodium, and meloxicam. Side effects include stomach distress.
- Analgesics: acetaminophen.
- Gabapentin.
- Opioids: tramadol, hydrocodone-containing drugs, and morphine sulfate. Side effects include sedation and constipation. Respiratory depression is not felt to be significant in the setting of treating pain.

How Can I Treat Depression?

Depression is not common in ALS, but it needs to be recognized when present (see Chapter 6). It is important to consider whether the patient has experienced (and has been treated for) depression in the past. Most importantly, if there is a question of "reduced mood," mood-elevating medications should be offered. A large selection of medications are available and are listed with their doses in Table 13–8; the choice is influenced by whether the patient has used one to good effect in the past and by minor features of each one:

- Selective serotonin reuptake inhibitors (SSRIs): fluoxetine, sertraline, paroxetine, citalopram, and bupropion. Common side effects include drowsiness or agitation and loss of libido.
- Amitriptyline: Used in ALS patients to manage many symptoms; doses for these purposes are lower than those to treat depression but may still have an effect on mood. Common side effects include dry mouth and constipation.

TABLE 13–8 Medications Used to Treat Reduced Mood and Depression

Medication	How Supplied	Uses	Preparation	Crushable	Dosage	Frequency	Side Effects
Amitriptyline (Elavil)	Prescription	Pseudobulbar affect Saliva control Sleep aid	Tablet	Yes	25 to 50 mg	At night	Anticholinergic
Bupropion (Wellbutrin)	Prescription	Mood Depression	Tablet IR Tablet XL	Yes No	100 mg 150 mg	2 times daily Daily	
Citalopram (Celexa)	Prescription	Mood Depression	Tablet, solution	Yes	20 to 40 mg	1 daily	
Fluoxetine (Prozac)	Prescription	Mood Depression	Tablet	Yes	20 to 80 mg	1 daily	
Paroxetine (Paxil)	Prescription	Mood Depression	Tablet, solution	No	20 to 40 mg	1 daily	
Sertraline (Zoloft)	Prescription	Mood Depression	Tablet	Yes	50 to 200 mg	1 daily	

How Can I Treat Anxiety?

Anxiety is an emotional state, and in the setting of ALS, anxiety can include a component of panic. It is frequently associated with a feeling of shortness of breath, which usually lasts only minutes and therefore may not indicate actual serious difficulty with breathing. The first episode is the most frightening. For some patients, subsequent episodes are less severe, and caregivers can help by providing soothing support. However, since panic attacks are distressing, it is appropriate to treat them. The most appropriate medication is a short-acting benzodiazepine like the following medications; doses are listed in Table 13–9:

- Clonazepam: A common side effect is sedation.
- Lorazepam: A common side effect is sedation.

How Can I Get Better Sleep?

Many people, both those with and those without ALS, describe their sleep as poor, having either difficulty falling asleep or difficulty returning to sleep after awakening in the middle of the night. One question to ask is whether a person's sleep is "restorative." In other words, was the person sufficiently rested to be able to stay awake and be alert during the day and into the evening? Indications that sleep is not restorative include falling asleep at work or at home when one wants to be awake and not being able to stay awake to watch television or read in the evening. Everyone has an occasional bad night, but if a person can manage daily activities, their sleep is doing the job. For the patient with ALS who cannot be physically active at work or in the home, maintaining attention may be difficult, and patients may fall asleep during the day.

If sleep is a concern, a number of factors should be considered. The most important is whether weakness of the diaphragm

TABLE 13-9 Medications Used to Treat Anxiety

Medication	How Supplied	Uses	Preparation	Crushable	Dosage	Frequency	Side Effects
Clonazepam (Klonopin)	Prescription	Anxiety	Tablet	Yes	0.25 mg	As needed	Sedation
Lorazepam (Ativan)	Prescription	Anxiety Pain	Tablet	Yes	1 to 2 mg	As needed	Sedation

is resulting in disturbed sleep that does not make the patient feel restored in the morning (see Chapter 6). The next most important factor is sleep hygiene, which means spending a reasonable amount of time in bed to sleep and not taking naps during the day. The average need for sleep is approximately 8 hours. If a patient uses 2 hours of their sleep allocation with a nap, then he or she may need only 6 hours more sleep and may feel frustrated when lying awake at night.

Patients far along with ALS may be worried about their course and future. Anxiety can be high, especially at night when the day's distractions are out of mind and a person turns inward. It is important for such patients to discuss issues that weigh on their mind and try to address them before going to sleep.

Many medications are advertised to help sleep. While they are effective, their improvement in sleep time is modest, about 15 minutes, and it is usually recommended that they be used only for short periods of time when a particular issue is causing the disturbed sleep. While practices vary among ALS clinics, these medications are not generally recommended for ALS patients. However, they should be discussed if other efforts are not successful. The following medications and their doses are listed in Table 13–10:

- Melatonin
- Amitriptyline
- Diphenhydramine
- Trazodone

A 5- to 6-ounce glass of wine in the evening may also help with sleep.

What If I Can't Swallow Pills?

Many medications to treat symptoms are pills (tablets or capsules). Swallowing pills taxes the coordination of swallowing muscles,

TABLE 13-10 Medications Used to Treat Disturbed Sleep

Medication	How Supplied	Uses	Preparation	Crushable	Dosage	Frequency	Side Effects
Amitriptyline (Elavil)	Prescription	Pseudobulbar affect Saliva control Sleep aid	Tablet	Yes	25 to 50 mg	At night	Anticholinergic
Diphenhydramine (Benadryl)	Over the counter	Sleep aid	Tablet, solution	Yes	25 to 50 mg	At night	Sedation
Melatonin	Over the counter	Sleep aid	Tablet	No	1 to 3 mg	At night	Sedation
Trazodone	Prescription	Sleep aid	Tablet	Yes	25 to 50 mg	At night	

as the water taken with pills passes through rapidly but the pills travel more slowly. With ALS, coordination of swallowing muscles is impaired, and pills may get caught on the way through. Some medications can be crushed and some cannot. Those that cannot be crushed can be swallowed more easily in a spoonful of applesauce or yogurt. Those that can be crushed can be mixed with water and swallowed. Some medications are available in a liquid form. If a patient is using a gastric feeding tube, medications that can be crushed or are in liquid form can be delivered through the tube. The tables in this chapter include listings of which medications can or cannot be crushed and which are available in liquid form.

Chapter 14

The Caregiver and ALS

When the diagnosis of ALS is made, the caregiver is the next most affected person after the patient, followed by (other) family members. The caregiver soon realizes that he or she will be responsible for providing greater amounts of care over time as the patient becomes weaker and less able to manage daily activities. The increased demands will decrease the caregiver's personal time and will sometimes create financial burdens as well. Caregivers will be confronted with both the physical burden of providing care and the emotional burden from the sadness of watching the patient decline and lose independence. There is also the realization that ultimately the patient will pass away and, if the caregiver is the patient's partner, that he or she will be alone. The increasing physical and emotional burdens can be compounded if the patient has elements of FTLD.

During clinic visits, most thoughts and efforts focus on the patient, but it is also important to address caregiver burden and coping strategies. During clinic visits the neurologist, nurse, or social worker should inquire after the caregiver. Caregivers should always raise their concerns during clinic visits if not asked. Support groups are another venue for caregivers to get help with their questions and challenges.

Who Provides Care?

Every ALS patient will need someone to provide care as the weakness progresses. ALS affects adults, and thus most caregivers are spouses, although children, other relatives, neighbors, or friends sometimes fill this role. Sometimes it takes a combination of family and friends. The most important characteristics for a caregiver are the willingness and ability to provide care. Willingness to provide care, not only for the family but for others, is part of human nature, and usually more help is offered than is actually accepted.

It is rare that an ALS patient needs care in a nursing home. However, patients and caregivers may benefit from health aides coming into the home several times a week to assist with bathing and dressing. This service can free the caregiver for rest or to perform other necessary activities. Patients may be reluctant to have another person bathe them, since this exposes part of their personal space (figuratively and literally). Caregivers may feel inadequate if another individual carries out the activities they consider their personal duty to their partners. These are issues that can be discussed with the neurologist and social worker.

How Does Providing Care Change with ALS Progression?

As the patient becomes weaker, the caregiver will have more to do. The order depends upon which area was affected first by ALS, but with time most areas are affected, and the extent of weakness at late stages requires total care.

With onset in the bulbar region, speech and communication will likely become a significant problem early on, and care efforts focus on trying to understand speech. At the same time, swallowing becomes problematic, and helping the patient sustain nutritional needs becomes an issue.

With onset in the arms, progressive help with bathing, dressing, and personal hygiene will be needed. If the arms are markedly weak, assistance with feeding will be needed.

With onset in the legs, assisting with bathing, dressing, and transfers and helping with changes in position in the middle of the night become issues.

Furthermore, the level of care is always changing. Once a routine is established for providing a certain level of care, the patient's needs may increase, and the level of care must be modified or changed. This happens again and again.

The caregiver must often accomplish patient care while keeping the household running. This can be particularly difficult when small children are part of the family or when the caregiver is working. There is also the psychological issue of keeping a strong front while ALS progresses.

The sum of all these difficulties is often labeled "caregiver burden."

What Is the Best Way to Offer Help?

The need for care should be viewed from the perspective of both patient and caregiver. The patient is frustrated with daily tasks that he or she previously performed without thought and now finds to be harder or even unmanageable. Patients often do not want to ask for assistance because of pride and other issues, while the caregiver often sees the patient struggling and wants to help. It is also common that the caregiver does not want to accept help from others, instead preferring to shoulder the entire caregiver burden alone. As a result, help may not be readily accepted by either the patient or the caregiver, and stress can increase for both parties. This pattern can repeat and become even more apparent as weakness progresses and both patient and caregiver need more help.

An approach to reducing patient and caregiver stress around the issue of help is to periodically take time to "negotiate" what types of help are needed and when. Setting aside a time for this can reduce emotions that arise at moments of crisis. Such negotiations will need to be repeated periodically as more help is needed. It may be helpful to involve other family members who can lend support.

> John had a can-do personality before ALS, and he was also stubborn. When weakness from ALS made him dependent upon others for simple daily activities, he did not easily accept help. This frustrated his wife, Carol, and other family members. One approach that was successful was for Carol to call a family meeting and ask everyone to share their concerns with John and assure him that even though he was capable of doing many things for himself, they would like to help him with some activities. Carol also asked John to explain what he wanted to continue to try to do to retain his autonomy, and the family then knew how to support him. The family continued to meet as a unit every other Sunday.

How Do Patients and Caregivers Manage?

As challenging new issues arise during the course of ALS, how the patient and caregiver managed stressful issues before the onset of ALS becomes an important factor. If their previous coping skills were successful and well established, their approach to new issues related to ALS will likely follow suit. Most partners gladly rise to the occasion, and there are examples of divorced spouses coming forward to help when the patient had been living alone. If previous coping skills were not successful, new issues may be problematic. Children can also help, but they frequently have their own families and work schedules that limit their availability.

When stressful situations pile up, it is useful to seek help in sorting them out. All stressful situations in life can benefit from counseling. The goal of counseling is to understand how individuals feel about the situation and how to mesh disparate feelings in a constructive manner. Many families experiencing ALS have not previously turned to counseling when other issues arose; thus patients and caregivers may need encouragement to consider counseling related to the challenges of ALS. In our ALS clinic the social worker inquires about possible stressful issues.

How Do Caregivers Manage Changes in Roles?

When one member of a couple develops ALS, changes will occur in roles that have become traditional over the duration of the relationship. The roles can be obvious or subtle. Obvious ones are who manages finances, makes home and automobile repairs, cares for the yard, or manages children. Subtle ones are who manages household chores, makes appointments, and so forth. For some roles, the change in who performs the role is straightforward, but for others it can require gaining new information, getting access to resources, and learning new skills and routines that the patient previously managed, such as paying bills or simple home repairs.

Every role the patient gives up must be assumed by the caregiver or another person. The change does not always go smoothly. Patients may feel inadequate because they cannot manage what they could in the past, and they may be reluctant to give up past responsibilities. Frequently, past experiences in the relationship predict how smoothly the changes will be made. Both parties should acknowledge the difficulties of having to take on and give up traditional roles. Formally sitting down to negotiate how the changes will be carried out can be helpful.

What Can Caregivers Do to Ease Their Care Burden?

As the burden of providing care increases, it is possible to have aides come into the home to help with the patient's bathing and dressing. Such aid is often scheduled three to five times a week, usually in the morning. Aid is frequently provided through hospice services (see Chapter 15).

If personal finances permit, having someone come in to clean the house or perform other chores on a regular basis can reduce the burden for the caregiver of maintaining the household. Adult children and neighbors can also be enlisted to help with shopping, errands, taking care of the yard, and other chores.

Note that many caregivers are used to managing the household without help, and they may perceive having outside people clean the house or run errands as casting doubt on their ability to manage. It is important to understand that during this time when the caregiver is under stress providing care for the patient, it is entirely appropriate to have outside help both in managing the household chores and in providing care.

Does Providing Care Affect Caregivers' Health?

Providing care is physically taxing. Caregivers can become sleep deprived if they have to attend to the patient during the night. Chronic sleep deprivation can worsen preexisting medical conditions and can to lead to accidents due to sleepiness. It is recommended that caregivers be given "care holidays" with a quiet night's sleep on a regular basis while someone else attends to the patient. Breaks of this sort, called **respites**, are discussed more later in the chapter.

Caregivers may have preexisting medical conditions that require treatment but that may be neglected because of the demands of caring for the ALS patient. General medical evaluations by the caregiver's primary care provider are recommended, perhaps twice yearly, or more frequently when the caregiver's symptoms worsen or new ones appear.

Caregivers may sustain injuries when transferring a patient, particularly if the patient slips and falls and brings down the caregiver.

Instruction on safe transfers by the clinic's physical therapist is essential, with periodic reviews as the patient becomes weaker.

What Do Caregivers Really Feel?

Helping and giving care to someone close has intrinsic rewards. However, negative feelings can also exist on a number of levels, some of which a caregiver would never express and may not want to acknowledge. The deepest set of feelings may be very raw and would involve "blue" language if expressed. While it is unwise to let these feelings surface, they are common and valid. One constructive way to defuse them is to work them out during physical exercise. Another way is to discuss them with a counselor.

Is Depression Common among Caregivers?

It is expected that providing care to an ALS patient will affect the caregiver's mood. While most of the time it does not cause a clinical depression, it can. If the caregiver is feeling overwhelmed and neither a brief respite nor talking to a friend helps, then it is time to seek counseling and possibly ask about a medication that can elevate mood. Caregiver depression likely reflects the situation, and the condition may lift after the patient passes away (though it may then be replaced with other emotions). Thus mood-elevating medications can realistically be considered to be temporary for the caregiver.

How Can a Caregiver Manage Stress?

There are a number of strategies that caregivers can try to manage stress, and their effectiveness will vary from person to person and from time to time. One is for the caregiver to be open to the patient, family, and ALS clinic personnel (nurse, neurologist, social worker) about the stresses he or she is experiencing. A second is periodic negotiations with the patient and family about the current needs of the patient and caregiver's ability to meet them. A third is for the caregiver to attend an ALS support group to vent frustrations and share strategies. A fourth is to get home health aides to assist with bathing and dressing the patient several times per week and to obtain household help to free up some time for the caregiver. A fifth is to organize periodic breaks (respites), such as walks, lunch with friends, or a weekend away. Family members or friends can help with care during these breaks.

Some caregivers have working careers that must be managed despite the need to provide more care in the home. It is taxing to work full-time at anything, but work outside the home can also offer a break from providing care. Nevertheless, as care needs increase over time, managing both work and patient care schedules can become difficult. At some point, a caregiver should consider a family medical leave (see Chapter 16).

What Are Respites?

Respites are periods of rest or relief from providing care. They can be as short as hours, allowing breathing space to attend to personal issues; somewhat longer, as with an uninterrupted night's sleep away from a patient who requires care at night; or longer still, as with a vacation of a weekend or more. Others can help with care during respites, and some state agencies and the ALS Association can assist with the costs of patient care during longer respites.

It is very important that a caregiver plan respites early in the course of providing care so that they are in place when really needed. This takes planning and help from people who may include family, friends, neighbors, and members of one's religious congregation.

Some agencies, such as hospice and state programs, provide for respite care. The clinic social worker can help identify such sources.

What Is Bereavement While the Patient Is Alive?

Bereavement is a response to a loss, which obviously occurs when a person dies. However, the bereavement process for both patient and caregiver can start early in the course of ALS, as they experience losses from the outset. The caregiver may mourn the loss of routine activities with the patient because the patient is weak and cannot participate in them. The caregiver may also mourn because providing care is restricting his or her normal outside activities. These are important issues for the caregiver to acknowledge and discuss, as they can foster resentment, which may be harder to manage at the time of the patient's death. A social worker or counselor can be helpful in exploring these issues.

Can a Caregiver Have Survivor's Guilt?

Survivor's guilt can take different forms. Why did the patient get sick and not me—especially when the patient has more to offer than I do? How will I survive without the patient being there? These are natural responses to a life-shortening illness. The clinic social worker or a counselor can help the caregiver sort through these feelings.

How Should the Caregiver Prepare for Being Alone?

Following the patient's death, the caregiver faces two main issues, one emotional and the other practical. The emotional issue is bereavement. This is a natural emotion, and dealing with it can be aided by attending bereavement groups or at least talking to someone. One never fully gets over the loss of a close family member, but there is a healing process over time.

The practical issue is management of financial affairs, some aspects of which are discussed in Chapter 16. It is important for the caregiver to learn about all ongoing financial issues. This is best managed slowly and early in the course of ALS.

Chapter 15

The End Stages of ALS

ALS is a progressive disorder. Eventually fewer and fewer lower motor neurons going to the diaphragm are left and breathing becomes insufficient, which causes death from respiratory failure. It is important to know that nothing in ALS happens suddenly, and each patient has his or her own rate of progression. Breathing difficulties increase slowly over a long period of time. An early sign of respiratory weakness is reduced breath support when speaking long sentences. Later there is difficulty with breathing comfortably when lying flat in bed, and the patient may require elevation of the head of the bed. At this stage, noninvasive ventilation is recommended (see Chapter 10). Patients may go from using noninvasive ventilation only at night to using it during naps, and eventually they may need it all the time. Occasionally patients will describe episodes lasting for several minutes of sudden "air hunger," a feeling of not being able to take in sufficient breath, even when they are sitting and are not active. These short-lived episodes are more likely due to anxiety or laryngeal spasms than to respiratory failure, because they are so brief.

How Do People with ALS Die?

The ALS patient dies from respiratory failure. With fewer lower motor neurons going to the diaphragm, diaphragm contractions become weaker and less carbon dioxide is eliminated, resulting in higher carbon dioxide levels in the blood. This causes mental fogginess and sedation. More shallow breathing can increase atelectasis, further reducing the passage of oxygen into the blood. In order for there to be adequate exchange of oxygen and carbon dioxide there must be adequate blood flow through the lungs and to other organs, which comes from the heart. At the end, when breathing becomes very slow, reduced oxygen in the blood supply to the heart becomes insufficient for the heart to function. At this point the heart stops and the patient dies. It may be somewhat comforting to know that high carbon dioxide causes mental fogginess and sedation, so the patient is not aware of this process.

Another factor in a patient's death can be dehydration. When ALS patients are close to the ends of their lives they may drink less, because they are less interested or because it is difficult to take in fluids without choking. Of note, people in their last few days of life do not desire fluids, and family members should not feel compelled to force fluids on them.

A third factor is that because the patient often becomes less mobile as the disorder progresses, blood flow to the limbs lessens as the body automatically preserves blood flow to internal organs. As a consequence of this reduced blood flow and of the lack of fluids in the body, blood clots may develop in veins in the legs that can move into the lungs and block the exchange of oxygen and carbon dioxide between the blood and the air in the lungs.

A fourth factor during the final days is the development of pneumonia due to poor respiratory effort, difficulties with swallowing secretions, and a weak cough.

Each patient will have other unique associated factors, including any chronic and ongoing disorders present before the onset of ALS. It is most important to know that death in ALS is usually peaceful, and that hospice care is there to ensure this is the case. The majority of patients with ALS in the United States die at home.

Although Diane was not planning to visit her parents that particular weekend, she sensed Lois was not doing well, so she rounded up Lois's twin, Lorene, and made an unscheduled trip. At that time Lois had begun sleeping in a recliner in the living room with Ray on the sofa at her side. Lois was tired but in good spirits and after the usual evening routine asked Diane to give her a manicure before she went to sleep. Lois died quietly that night. Ray, Lorene, and Diane were surprised at how peaceful that last evening had been.

What If I Want to Continue Living?

Although the natural course of ALS is for patients to pass away from respiratory failure, the patient can chose to use noninvasive or invasive ventilation that will support respiration when the diaphragm is too weak. With progression of ALS, patients are usually first offered noninvasive ventilation at night, as there is greater difficulty with breathing during sleep. Later, patients may feel the need to use noninvasive ventilation during the day, and eventually they may feel that they need it all of the time. With newer types of ventilator machines, some people can be maintained for long periods of time (up to 24 hours per day) using noninvasive ventilation. For other patients the air pressure needed to help breathing is so high that the mask used in noninvasive ventilation must be tight enough around the face to prevent leaks. In that case, the patient may choose to switch to invasive (tracheal) ventilation, which allows sufficient air to be delivered without the discomfort of the mask.

When respiratory function declines to the point that the patient needs invasive ventilation, the patient has the choice of whether to use the device or to be made comfortable and allowed to pass away. If the patient chooses some form of full-time ventilation, his or her breathing will be comfortable, but progressive weakening of muscles will continue throughout the body (see Chapter 10).

What If I Can't Make Up My Mind about Ventilation?

Deciding whether to use full-time ventilation to prolong life is a major and frightening question. It is understandable that a patient may be uncertain. It is important for a patient to discuss his or her thoughts and concerns with the caregiver and other family members. The issue may arise unexpectedly during a respiratory episode, in which case the decision to start ventilation may be made simply because no one knows the patient's wishes. The decision to use full-time ventilation will dramatically affect the caregiver, since around-the-clock care will now be required. It is important for the patient to acknowledge that full-time ventilation will increase the caregiver's burden, and it may be necessary to add additional caregivers. Chapter 10 discusses ways to manage a patient's decision not to use supported ventilation.

Betty began having difficulty with shortness of breath at night and initially benefited from using bilevel ventilation for this problem. Several months later she began using it during naps, and finally she did not feel comfortable breathing without it. Her neurologist and pulmonologist discussed invasive ventilation with her and asked whether she wanted it, but Betty could not decide. One afternoon she became acutely short of breath, and her husband, Henry, called 911. Emergency services took her to the hospital, where the doctors in the emergency department intubated her with an endotracheal tube to maintain her breathing. She had pneumonia, which was treated with

(Continued)

(Continued)

antibiotics, but when it cleared up, she could not breathe on her own. Since Betty and Henry had not previously discussed her wishes in detail and it was difficult to communicate with her, it was not possible to determine her wishes in this circumstance. As a result, she had a tracheostomy and ultimately went home with invasive ventilation. Henry, their children, and several friends trained to care for her. After 2 months at home, Betty wanted to be taken off the ventilator and pass away in peace. Hospice services came to the house, and with the family present, she was given medications to ensure her comfort, the ventilator was turned down, and she died in a natural manner.

What If I Don't Want to Continue Living?

If patients do not want supported ventilation, doctors and nurses can make them comfortable so they can pass away peacefully. If a patient initially choses invasive ventilation, a time will usually come when the patient has completed what he or she hoped for with the extra time and will want to be taken off the ventilation.

It is the role of hospice care to ensure a peaceful death in this situation. Medications can be given to reduce anxiety and discomfort and make the patient sleepy. With these medications, the patient drifts into sleep, the ventilator is turned down, and the patient passes away comfortably.

Do Patients with ALS Take Their Own Lives?

This is a difficult question to answer, for several diverse reasons. First, patients with any progressive disease such as ALS likely have thoughts at some time that they do not want to live with the disease.

There are no data on how many patients with ALS actively shorten their lives, but the number is likely small, because these thoughts are often fleeting and involve no solid wish to act on them. Later in the disease the patient may not have the physical means to take his or her own life. Legal restraints on enlisting help from a physician to actively bring about premature death vary by state in the United States and by country in other regions of the world. Research supports the idea that only a small number of patients with ALS die with physician assistance. The concept of patient autonomy, which concerns a patient's right to make decisions about his or her own care, includes the important and controversial issue of the patient's ability to "die with dignity" and to choose to shorten his or her life. The overriding concern is that a wish to die may reflect depression, which can be treated. It is most important that if a patient has actively given thought to shortening his or her life, these thoughts should be shared with the neurologist.

What Are Palliative and Hospice Care?

The goal of palliative care is to improve quality of life in the setting of a serious illness that predictably shortens a patient's life. Hospice care provides relief of symptoms when a patient has about 6 months to live. Palliative care and hospice care are usually combined, with the same group of doctors, nurses, and aides. The palliative care team can be introduced early in the clinic to reassure the patient and family that it will be there when needed. The palliative care team, along with ALS clinic personnel, can lay out the types of documents everyone needs when diagnosed with a progressive illness, including a power of attorney for medical care and personal finances (see Chapters 10 and 16).

Since the direct symptoms of ALS are limited to weakness, the focus of hospice services is to provide aid in the home with bathing and dressing. Once on hospice care, the patient should still consider attending ALS clinic appointments. However, when the patient is no longer able to go to the clinic, hospice services include nursing visits to inform the hospice doctor or the ALS clinic about any new issues. The hospice team can also provide emotional support to the caregiver and family, as it includes a social worker and clergy. Most importantly, hospice care can ensure that the patient passes away in comfort.

In the United States hospice care is funded by Medicare hospice benefits, and hospice assumes all costs of care. However, these funds are limited, and hospice cannot pay for procedures and expensive equipment. For ALS, procedures such as placement of a gastric feeding tube and equipment such as noninvasive ventilation and power wheelchairs are necessary to maintain quality of life. They can be used when the patient is on hospice care; however, hospice cannot pay for them. In our ALS clinic we review future needs for such equipment when hospice care is being considered. Even after hospice care has begun it may be possible to briefly leave hospice care, go back on general Medicare insurance to have procedures performed or equipment obtained, and then go back on hospice care.

When Should Hospice Care Be Considered?

Hospice care is recommended at late stages of ALS. If a patient does not wish to use supported ventilation to prolong life, hospice physicians and ALS physicians can make him or her comfortable and allow the patient to pass away without distress. If a patient was on supported ventilation and wants to be taken off, hospice personnel can be brought in. Note that when a patient is dependent upon invasive ventilation and plans to use it long term, hospice care cannot be used, because, as discussed in Chapter 10, hospice care is really for the last 6 months of life. When the patient wants to stop invasive ventilation, hospice care becomes available.

How Can Spirituality Help?

Spirituality is a broad term that includes a sense of connection to something bigger than oneself. It can be part of organized religion or a personal set of feelings. Some people participate in spiritual activities throughout their lives and on a regular basis, as by attending religious services. Most people think about where they fit into the larger picture when death is approaching. The concept of the larger picture may be well established within an individual or may be re-explored at this time. Clergy may also become important at this time, and if a patient has no identified individual in this role, hospice care usually includes spiritual counselors.

Chapter 16

Planning Ahead

Because ALS follows a progressive course and issues do not arise suddenly, a patient has time to discuss and arrange for medical care, arrange financial affairs, and complete estate planning.

Who Should I Tell?

ALS is not an invisible disease, and everyone who comes in contact with the patient will know something has changed. People who are not told about the diagnosis or who are unfamiliar with ALS may wrongly attribute speech difficulties and spastic gait to alcohol intoxication.

It is wise to tell every family member of the diagnosis of ALS. Members who come into contact with you will know something is happening; members who are remote may feel slighted when they learn of it at a later time. When ALS is diagnosed, it is time to be with family. If there are strained relationships, there is time to heal them.

Discussions with friends and neighbors are important also, as they can help when future needs arise. Employers should know they will have to fill work positions when weakness requires a patient to stop work activities, and will have to assist the patient with obtaining work-related health and disability insurance. Many people informed about the diagnosis may not know much about ALS, and having a brief description to hand out can be helpful. Such descriptions are available on the web pages of the Muscular Dystrophy

Association and the ALS Association. Our ALS clinic provides a very brief description of ALS on a business card to be carried next to the patient's driver's license.

How and What Should I Tell My Family?

There is no ideal way to tell your family about a serious diagnosis, and much depends upon the ages and geographic distribution of family members. One method is to gather together as many family members who live close by as possible and include more remote members by speaker telephone or Skype, so that everyone can share in the conversation.

Family members should receive a full account of ALS, including the prognosis. (What to tell young children is a special problem, discussed in the next section.) Having written information available is helpful; sources include the diagnostic clinic visit and reliable Internet sites like those of the MDA and ALSA. Questions should be written down and asked of the ALS clinic's nurse or at the next clinic visit. Family members should be cautioned that what they read on the Internet may not directly apply to "their" ALS patient.

What Should I Tell My Children?

ALS cannot be made invisible, and the diagnosis cannot be hidden from young children, who have an amazing ability to detect when something is changing. Unless they are given guidance, children will form their own thoughts about what is happening. Accordingly, patients are encouraged to initially acknowledge that they are having difficulties that are being evaluated. If the child asks to know more about the condition, let him or her know that it is of concern and explain that there is an unknown medical cause. It is important to explain in sufficient detail that the child is not at fault. As disabilities progress, it is good to find activities that the patient and child can participate in. When ALS reaches a critical point, it is important that the child understand that the patient will die from ALS.

A serious illness leading to death of a parent is a major challenge for children. In addition to keeping them informed, it may be beneficial to use religious beliefs to help the children cope. If a child appears not to be managing, the ALS clinic's social worker can be helpful, as can bereavement groups for children.

Older children have more experience with life. They can be informed early on that the parent may have a serious illness, and when the diagnosis is made it should be fully disclosed to older children. Most clinics welcome children attending the clinic visits. Many children ask about possible hereditary aspects of ALS, and this issue should be addressed with them. If there is a family history of ALS, a genetic counselor can be helpful (see Chapter 4).

What Are Medical Directives?

Medical directives are documents that communicate a person's decisions about medical care and are used only when the individual cannot effectively make his or her own medical decisions. Although most people with ALS are usually able to make decisions until their death, there are circumstances where advance directives are necessary. For example, if a patient has sudden respiratory failure and is not revived until after a brain injury has occurred or if the patient has lapsed into a coma, then it is unlikely that the patient will regain the ability to make competent decisions. In this type of situation, it is important for the family to know what the patient desired in order to implement those wishes.

There are several types of advance directives, some of which are described below. Their use is governed by laws and regulations in individual states. It is important that a patient become familiar with the documents used in his or her state.

Living Will

A **living will** is a written document that allows a person to indicate his or her wishes about healthcare, including end-of-life decisions. Most issues for ALS patients involve when to be resuscitated and whether to be intubated. Like all advance directives, living wills are useful in circumstances where the patient no longer has the capacity or the ability to make his or her own decisions. Some states have a specific form that must be used for a living will.

Power of Attorney for Healthcare

Although a **power of attorney for healthcare** (also called a power of attorney for medical affairs) is also used when the patient no longer has the capacity or ability to make his or her own decisions, it is much different from a living will because it names a specific person who will make medical decisions as the agent for the patient when the patient can no longer do so. The specific circumstances in which the agent will act are specified in the document. The patient should discuss those circumstances with the agent in advance so that the patient's wishes will be implemented if the need arises. As with a living will, some states have a specific form that must be used for a power of attorney for healthcare.

Do-Not-Resuscitate Order

Patients with ALS should consider whether they wish to have a do-not-resuscitate order. To **resuscitate** means to revive a person who has lost consciousness, usually from respiratory or cardiac causes. If the ALS patient does not want to be resuscitated, the order should be readily available to instruct emergency medical providers (emergency services or emergency department doctors) if the patient becomes unconscious or otherwise cannot give instructions about whether he or she wants to be resuscitated. Without such a directive, it is often an emergency provider's obligation to take life-saving measures, such as resuscitating the patient and starting invasive ventilation, even though that may not be what the patient wants. The names of do-not-resuscitate order forms may vary among states, and some states may require a specific form.

All advance directives (the living will, power of attorney for healthcare, and do-not-resuscitate order) should be prepared and signed while the patient is able to communicate easily and is capable of making his or her own medical decisions. Copies should be provided to the patient's primary care physician and neurologist, and another copy should be placed where it will be immediately available to family members as well as emergency and hospital personnel.

What Do I Need to Know about Estate Planning?

Everyone should have an estate plan, yet many people avoid making one. Because ALS is a terminal disease, patients with ALS should create an estate plan if they do not already have one or update an existing estate plan if they do.

An **estate** consists of all a person's possessions, including favorite (and not so favorite) things, money, real estate, and inheritances, to name a few categories. An estate also includes life insurance and pension amounts payable on death.

An estate plan, like an advance directive, can include several kinds of documents, not all of which are appropriate for all people. Documents are based on laws in the state that the patient lives in. In general, these documents may include **wills**, **trusts**, and **powers of attorney for financial affairs**. An estate plan can even include lifetime gifts, putting property into joint tenancy, or payable-on-death accounts, as provided for by state law. Because property transfers can have adverse consequences (for example, with respect to taxes, unintended exposure to a transferee's creditors, and other matters), these alternatives should be discussed with an attorney before such transfers are made. If there are young children in the family, it may be necessary to name a guardian to look after their interests following the patient's death or incapacity.

Brief descriptions of the documents that may be used in an estate plan are provided below. The details given are appropriate in Utah at this time, but could change in future years as laws change and may be different in other states.

Will

A will is usually part of every estate plan. In basic terms, it is a legal document appointing a personal representative for the estate and instructing that representative to distribute specific assets to specific beneficiaries after the death of the patient. The will becomes effective at the time of death. When a person's assets total less than the current federal estate tax credit, a will may be the only document needed to deal with the estate. For more complex estates, a will is often used in combination with other estate-planning documents.

Trust Agreement

A trust agreement is a legal document in which a **trustee** is appointed to administer and distribute assets according to terms specified in the document. A trust should be considered for more complex estates, and the assets must be transferred into it before death. Trusts function much differently from wills because only the assets in the trust will be administered by the trustee. These assets will not be distributed under the will.

Power of Attorney for Financial Affairs

Powers of attorney can be very useful when another person needs to act on behalf of the patient. There are powers of attorney for both healthcare decisions (discussed above) and for financial affairs. A **power of attorney for financial affairs** designates a person to act as an agent in financial matters during the patient's lifetime. In some cases the agent is given very general directions and broad powers. In other situations the agent is specifically directed to act in a limited way and only as specified in the power of attorney.

Lifetime Gift

A person often has possessions that family members or friends would like to have. One way to ensure that those possessions are distributed as desired is to give them away during one's lifetime. Lifetime gifts have the added benefit of allowing the giver and the recipients to enjoy the giving and receiving process while avoiding strife among family members and friends at death if more than one person wants a particular item. It is reasonable for people to consider who would like what possessions and to plan to pass those items on during their lifetime in order to enjoy the gifting process.

> John could build and fix anything before his weakness from ALS began. He had one or more tools for every task. As John became too weak to use his favorite tools, he did not want them to gather dust in the garage and be discarded after his death. He decided to give specific tools to people who he knew would use them and appreciate that they were from him.

Estate planning will vary among people, and all but the simplest estates benefit from consultation with an attorney. If a person dies without an estate plan, the estate will be disbursed as set forth in the laws of the state in which the person resides. Thus if a person has particular items he or she wants to pass on to a particular individual, it is important to make that happen through an estate plan, by making sure that title is held in the desired manner or by making a lifetime gift. Everyone should complete an estate plan to avoid legal issues, questions, or misunderstandings after death. This is particularly true for people with ALS.

What about Computer Passwords and Safety Deposit Boxes?

Many financial transactions are managed through the Internet. In some families, one member manages the finances, and he or she may be the only person who knows passwords for computers and financial websites. If that person has ALS and dies without sharing those passwords, it can be very difficult to log into computers and gain access to those websites. Further, some families have safety deposit boxes containing documents that are needed after death, and it can be a lengthy process for the spouse or partner to gain access to the contents of such a box if it is not arranged prior to the patient's death.

What about Health Insurance?

Health insurance is important for anyone, and particularly so for someone with ALS, as optimal care may be expensive.

Medicare

ALS affects adults, and many patients have health insurance through their employment. In the United States, if a person has worked and paid taxes into Social Security and has earned a sufficient number of credits or quarters, he or she is eligible for Medicare total disability. The number of work quarters, the time for which the person has worked, and the person's age are relevant variables here. When a diagnosis of ALS is made, a patient should immediately notify the Social Security Administration to receive the most accurate information. At the time of this writing it takes 5 months from the date of diagnosis for Medicare health insurance to become effective.

If a person is working at the time of the ALS diagnosis and has health insurance through the employer, he or she should discuss the diagnosis with the employer's human resources department before applying for Medicare, as protocols may be in place for short- and long-term disability health insurance. If a person carries his or her own health insurance, he or she should contact the insurance company, to determine which is a better option.

Military Veteran Benefits

Persons diagnosed with ALS who served for at least 90 days in the US armed forces (Army, Marine Corps, Navy, Air Force, Coast Guard, and National Guard if called to active duty) are eligible for military service disability at the 100 percent disability rating. Military disability offers substantial benefits that include medications, equipment to enhance mobility (wheelchairs, lifts, ramps, handicapped vehicles), and home renovations. If the veteran has not been seen or has not recently been followed in a Veterans Administration Medical Center (VAMC) clinic or hospital, he or she needs to make an appointment to establish care and to receive benefits. Some VAMC facilities have specialty ALS clinics, but if the patient's particular facility does not, it is recommended that the patient continue with his or her ALS specialty clinic and have it recommend equipment needs to the VAMC clinic.

Should I Keep Working?

Whether to continue working is a personal question, but there are several issues to consider. For some people, work is important for self-esteem; for others, continuing to work hinders them from doing other, more enjoyable things. If the decision is to continue working, activities will become more challenging over time. Work safety should be considered if work requires physical activity with potential for falling or being injured by equipment. It is wise to discuss the diagnosis of ALS with managers and coworkers, as changes will be noticed and it may be important to find and train a replacement. The patient should also work with human resources on insurance benefits such as short- and long-term disability and the start of Medicare.

What Is Family and Medical Leave?

The Family and Medical Leave Act (FMLA) is a federal law from 2009 that allows for up to 12 weeks of unpaid, job-protected leave from work per year. Group health benefits are maintained during the leave. The program allows an individual to provide care for an immediate family member with a serious health condition for this period of time. FMLA applies to public agencies and companies with more than 50 employees and has other eligibility requirements. The caregiver should consult with the employer to determine whether FMLA applies to him or her.

FMLA can be used in a variety of ways, including providing periodic time to accompany the patient to clinic visits, time for family gatherings and holidays, respite for the primary caregiver, or just time to spend with the patient toward the end of the course of ALS.

What Are Other Financial Considerations?

A variety of financial issues and questions can arise in the setting of ALS that depend upon a patient's financial portfolio. These questions should be taken up with a financial manager. For patients who have a family business, an income threshold applies to Medicare. For those who have life insurance, there may be a payout in the setting of a terminal disorder while the patient is still living.

Chapter 17

Research in ALS

What Is Going On in ALS Research?

Every patient asks what is new in ALS research and when will a cure be discovered. There are perhaps two kinds of research in ALS: one is investigation into understanding causes, and the other involves finding effective drugs for the treatment of symptoms and causes. Investigations into causes are considered "laboratory bench science," and finding effective drugs is considered "clinical investigation." The pathway between these two types of research is called "bench to bedside." Both types of research are complex and time-consuming.

Research takes place in laboratories at universities or at pharmaceutical companies. There are a number of agencies that fund ALS research. In the United States, the National Institutes of Health (NIH) spent $44 million on ALS in 2015, the Muscular Dystrophy Association spent $500,000 in 2015, and the ALS Association received over $100 million from its Ice Bucket Challenge to be used over several years. The question is often asked whether even more money would hasten development of a cure. Unfortunately, the answer is likely no, as ALS is a difficult disease to unravel, and spending more money could lead to inefficient research. It is important to know that many research laboratories throughout the world focus all of their efforts on ALS. As mentioned in Chapter 1, there are similar challenges in understanding and treating all neurodegenerative diseases, but their similarities also mean that research on one is research on all of them.

In addition to discovering more effective drugs, research is also being conducted on coming up with medications to treat symptoms and understanding how ALS affects the lives of patients and caregivers.

How Are Drugs Discovered and Tested?

Drugs are selected to be tested because bench science research indicates that the drug might act at a site or sites in the proposed mechanisms of ALS (see Chapter 4). In the United States, all drugs must be approved by the US Food and Drug Administration (FDA), and in Europe they must be approved by the European Medicines Agency (EMA). A rigorous three-phase testing process ensures that a drug is safe (has no significant side effects) and effective (does what it is intended to do). Phase 1 drug trials are very small, with only a few subjects. Phase 2 trials are larger, with 20 to 100 subjects. Phase 3 trials are very large, with 300 to 600 subjects, and require multiple clinics (medical centers) to participate. Phase 3 trials are therefore called multicenter trials; they are also called the pivotal trials, as they are largely what the FDA relies upon to approve a drug. Ultimately, a cocktail of several drugs may be tested, each acting at a specific site.

Testing a drug for ALS takes many years. First, it takes several years to design a study. Once a trial is started, each subject is followed for 9 to 12 months. Shorter trials are less likely to show a slowing in the rate of ALS progression. Since phase 3 trials enroll 300 to 600 subjects, it generally takes at least 2 to 3 years between when the first subject starts and the last subject finishes, and then the data have to be analyzed before results are available.

A major challenge in an ALS drug trial is how to measure a positive effect. With progressive loss of upper and lower motor neurons, strength and function cannot be restored, making it difficult for a drug to show a slowing of the rate of progression. Because markedly different rates of progression exist among ALS patients, a large number of subjects are required to encompass the spectrum of rates (explaining the need for 300 to 600 subjects). ALS progression can be measured by patient survival (the measure used with the drug riluzole; see Chapter 7) or by the ALS Functional Rating Scale (see Chapter 5).

At this time, most drug trials for ALS include a group of control patients who receive a **placebo** (a sugar pill) to ensure that any evidence that the tested medication is really working is valid: if patients taking the medication do not improve compared with the placebo group, then the medication cannot be considered effective. Patients are randomly assigned to receive either the active drug or placebo, and everyone in the trial, including the researchers, is blinded as to who receives what. (The code is held by a special board overseeing the study and can be broken if needed.) Many patients are uncomfortable with the idea of being randomly assigned to a placebo, but there is no other rigorous way to ensure that the drug or intervention is truly having a positive effect. The concept of **equipoise** (equal balance) refers to researchers' assuming at the start of a trial that the drug being tested is as likely to be effective as it is to be ineffective or even harmful. The sponsors of the trial are comfortable with this balance, which gives the drug and the placebo an equal chance. Experience with a large number of drugs tested for ALS indicates that most showed no effect (equal balance) and some showed a worse outcome for those patients taking the active drug compared with those taking the placebo.

There is discussion about comparing rates of progression for patients receiving drugs currently being tested with those of placebo patients enrolled in past drug trials (historic controls). However, the general level of patient care may have improved between the old and new study, and historic placebo data may not be accurate. Another approach to avoiding the use of current placebo controls is to determine rates of progression for each subject for a few months at the beginning of the trial before starting the experimental drug and then to look for a change in progression after starting the drug. There is concern, however, that the disease state may be different early on compared with later on, and that the success of a drug might depend upon an early start.

ALS drug studies are very expensive, costing tens of millions of dollars. It is important to appreciate that well over 125 drug trials have been completed for ALS over the past 25 years, but unfortunately only riluzole has demonstrated any effect on the disease.

Where Can I Get More Information about Trials?

All drug trials for ALS are listed in the NIH website at www.clinical-trials.gov. Not all clinics participate in all trials, and patients should discuss current trials with the ALS clinic neurologist. Some clinics have their own research projects that do not involve taking medications but that provide useful information about ALS management and genetics.

Should I Participate in a Trial?

ALS patients are encouraged to participate in drug trials and other types of research projects. Participation helps us advance the understanding of ALS, find more drugs, and manage patients more effectively. Participation also allows patients to feel that they are actively involved with discovering new information. Participation in a drug trial requires time and effort on the part of the patient and caregiver, who must come to the clinic for study visits over a period of 9 to 12 months. Some research projects, such as completing a questionnaire, require less time. Patients and caregivers usually feel that the frequent contact with a neurologist while participating in a research study is a positive experience and worth the time and effort.

A patient who participates in a trial is unlikely to directly benefit from it, as trials take a number of years to complete. Thus neurologists who run trials appreciate the good faith about the future that each participating patient gives.

What Is Informed Consent?

To participate in a clinical trial, patients must be fully informed about the design of the trial, the procedures and obligations it entails, the tests to be performed, and the risks and benefits. It is essential that the patient fully understand these elements, so that they can then give their full consent to participating in the trial—hence the term "informed consent." However, since FTLD or elements of FTLD are present in approximately 50 percent of ALS patients, the question arises of how to guarantee full understanding. Every clinical trial has inclusion and exclusion criteria, and one inclusion criterion is the ability to understand the trial design. Usually the neurologist participating in the trial makes the determination of the ability of the patient to understand all aspects of the trial, including risks. In general, risks of drug trials have been small and unexpected side effects very rare. It is important that the caregiver inform the trial staff of his or her feelings about the patient's ability to understand what participation in the trial involves.

Let Me Try It—What Do I Have to Lose?

If a patient is not eligible for a drug trial or does not want to participate in one, he or she may say, "Let me try the drug—what do I have to lose?" Many states in the United States have enacted "right to try" bills allowing terminally ill patients to get access to experimental treatments. Such bills are modeled after a federal policy called "expanded access," also called "compassionate use" of experimental drugs. The idea is to give patients access to research drugs outside of clinical trials. A similar situation occurs when patients take unapproved treatments available on the Internet (such as stem cells).

There are several concerns with this approach. One is that the drug or treatment may be harmful or hasten the rate of disease progression, but this effect may not be obvious with a single "subject." A second is that with a single subject, it will be difficult to accurately determine if there is a slowing in progression, especially if the effect is modest, and moreover, since no information is formally collected, any positive effect will be of no help to future patients. A third is that the drug company may not be able to supply the experimental drug. Finally, treatment may be costly, because insurance may not pay for a drug that has not been approved for use in ALS.

There are many supplements and unregulated treatments available. Some insight as to their effectiveness can be obtained from patients who have taken them and have posted their experiences on the website patientslikeme.com.

Chapter 18

Concluding Thoughts

Neurologist's Perspective

There are few if any diseases more challenging than ALS for the patient, caregiver, and family. With life there is death. We know this from a young age, and we are reminded of the natural progression when family and friends die and from the media reporting on the deaths of people remote to us. There are occasional thoughts as to how we will die, whether from a disease yet to be diagnosed, unexpectedly, or in some other manner. ALS is unique in that for all involved the progression and manner of death are known to a reasonable degree. In some sense this can be an advantage, as plans can be made to reach closure with family and friends.

ALS is a disease of adults, and the distribution of the age of death from ALS is about 8 to 10 years earlier than that for the whole population from any cause. This is a sad number, but the ALS patient needs to be assured that there are many laboratories and efforts directed toward shortening this interval. The most common causes of death for everyone are heart disease and cancer. Heart disease can be a chronic condition limiting physical activities or can cause sudden death. Cancer is associated with treatment and remissions, which come along with the anxiety and rollercoaster uncertainty about whether remission will last or will be followed by an untreatable relapse.

In times of old, aging family members lived with their families, and their demise was part of family life. In current times, families are dispersed, work schedules are hectic, and the dying process has become somewhat sterile. The vast majority of ALS patients in the United States wish to die at home, and do so. The slow course of ALS allows for at least a partial return to a more natural process.

The challenges in ALS are large. For the patient and family there is the emotional and progressive pathway to death. For the patient there may be a spiritual component to this pathway. For all involved there are the physical challenges of managing daily activities, which can be eased only partially by technological innovations and equipment. Overriding these challenges is the innate desire of caregivers and family to help and the process for the patient of shifting priorities (response shift).

Caregiver burden increases over time and frequently becomes a 24-hour-a-day, 7-day-a-week job lasting months to years. Caregivers may maintain a visible smile but likely have very strong emotions below the surface. It has been observed that following the death of the patient caregivers move away from ALS rapidly and thoroughly. This is understandable, but the ALS community should provide specialized bereavement support. Many ALS clinics send a card acknowledging the loss. Some make a phone call, but the call usually comes right after the death, at the least opportune time for the caregiver. Some clinics have a yearly recognition of patients who have passed away during the year, a modification of a "yahrzeit," the Jewish tradition of honoring a loved one's passing and remembering him or her as a person on the anniversary of the death.

There is frustration among ALS researchers and neurologists that we still do not know what causes ALS nor do we have an effective medication to slow its course. The proposals for possible causes of ALS outlined in Chapter 4 remain theories, but the lack of a clear understanding has not stopped clinical drug trials, well over 125 of which have been conducted over the past 25 years. Unfortunately, these trials have been unsuccessful (with the partial exception of riluzole); still, they point out the efforts being made to increase survival.

As a neurologist who has given the diagnosis of ALS to a large number of patients and followed them in clinic over the past 30 years, I am impressed that patients so often handle their disease with grace. At the time of making the diagnosis, neurologists can predict the course and challenges that patients and families will face. Despite this foreknowledge, a survey of ALS neurologists about their feelings indicated that all were committed to the task of providing the best possible care based on the individual patient, caregiver, and family. All felt that it was a rewarding experience to be an ALS neurologist.

Caregiver's Perspective

The most difficult aspect of ALS for caregivers is that the ALS patient progresses to become almost totally physically dependent on the caregiver. Living with ALS begins with weakness that can be managed by the patient, but shifts to weakness that can only be managed with a great deal of physical assistance from caregivers. As the weakness progresses, so does the caregiver's desire and commitment to help, but caregivers should not hesitate to ask for and accept offers of help as their burden increases.

This steadily progressing physical weakness is one feature of ALS that distinguishes it from other terminal diseases. It can be a blessing that the progression and manner of death from ALS are somewhat predictable. This predictability gives all involved time to plan in many ways. By contrast, most people have known someone with cancer who has experienced the elation of being in remission, only to learn soon thereafter that the cancer has returned. The cancer patient rides a rollercoaster of hope.

The ALS patient who is able to stay emotionally engaged in living life can continue to share good times with the people in his or her life. Unless there is marked FTLD, this remains true until the end of life, as the limitations imposed by the disease are primarily physical, not mental or emotional. The patient is able to spend quality time with loved ones and friends, to check off things on his or her bucket list, and to rebuild or repair relationships that may have been neglected. Savoring life and being grateful for this time can bring joy and satisfaction. On the practical side of things, there is also time for patients to really think about how their possessions should be disposed of at death and to implement those decisions.

The family and caregiver also have time not only to say goodbye but to show the patient how much he or she is loved and appreciated. The simple act of caring for someone you love day after day speaks much louder than words.

GLOSSARY

Accessory muscles of respiration: Muscles that raise the shoulders and expand the ribcage and are used when short of breath, either from running or ALS, in contrast to the main muscle used during inhalation (the diaphragm).

Aggregates: In ALS, clumps of proteins in nerve cells that may be toxic to cells.

Air stacking: A breathing exercise to increase lung volume in which one repeatedly adds or stacks one small inhalation upon another to maximally expand the lungs. Also called breath stacking.

ALS Functional Rating Scale–Revised (ALSFRS-R): A clinical assessment of a patient's global ability to function that is also used as a measure of disease progression in the clinic and in ALS drug studies.

Amalgam: The filing dentists use to fill teeth after decayed areas have been removed. Also known as silver fillings.

Amyotrophic: Marked by atrophy, or shrinkage, of muscles due to loss of lower motor nerves going to the muscle.

Ankle-foot orthosis (AFO): A brace across the ankle that holds the foot at a right angle to the lower leg to reduce catching the toe when walking.

Anticholinergic side effects: Side effects of certain medications that block the function of the neurotransmitter acetylcholine in the autonomic nervous system.

Atelectasis: Closure or collapse of air sacs in the lung, resulting in reduced gas exchange.

Atrophy: Shrinkage of muscle due to loss of lower motor neurons.

Autonomic nervous system: Portion of the nervous system that controls heart rate and blood pressure, the digestive system, and body temperature (as by sweating and constriction of blood vessels).

Autonomy: The right of a patient to make his or her own medical decisions.

Autosomal dominant: Inheritance pattern where only one copy of an abnormal gene (mutation) needs to be present in an individual for the disease to develop.

Autosomal recessive: Inheritance pattern where two copies of an abnormal gene (mutation) need to be present in an individual for the disease to develop.

Bilevel noninvasive ventilation: Form of assisted ventilation in which the ventilator gives more air with each breath than the patient can inhale alone. "Bilevel" refers to the use of two levels of pressure, high for inhalation and lower for exhalation. BiPAP is a brand name of a device for bilevel noninvasive ventilation.

Body mass index (BMI): A measure of the body that takes into account both weight and stature (height).

Bone marrow stem cells: Partially differentiated stem cells obtained from bone marrow.

Brain-computer interface: A device that uses brainwaves recorded with electrodes on the scalp to control a marker on a computer that can be used to spell out words.

Brainstem: The portion of the brain between the cerebral hemispheres and the spinal cord.

Breath stacking: See *air stacking*.

Bulbar region: Portion of the brainstem where upper motor neurons control lower motor neurons that activate muscles for speech and swallowing; it gets its name because it looks like a tulip bulb.

Carbon dioxide: Waste product of energy production in all cells; accumulates in the blood, is removed in the lungs, and leaves the body in exhaled air.

Catheter: A thin tube that is inserted into the body and drains fluid to the outside of the body.

Central fatigue: A feeling of fatigue out of proportion to muscle weakness or sleepiness.

Cerebral cortex: Main, outer part of the brain. It is divided into lobes such as the frontal and temporal lobes. Also called the cerebral hemispheres.

Cervical spine region: The neck, including the bony spine (vertebrae) and a portion of the spinal cord.

Chelation: Binding of a toxic substance to a carrier drug so that it can be removed from the body.

Chromosomes: Structures within a cell that contain DNA and the genetic code.

Cluster: Group of people with a high rate of ALS who live or lived in a small geographical region.

Conduction block: Rare condition where motor nerve impulses are blocked at a focal point along a nerve, resulting in weakness without degeneration of lower motor nerve fibers.

CoughAssist device: A mechanical device that enhances the power of a cough.

Deep venous thrombosis (DVT): A blood clot in a deep-lying vein in a leg or arm.

Dementia: Disorder of mental processing.

Diaphragm: Main muscle used for breathing.

Dietitian: Healthcare provider who assesses nutritional needs and suggests how to achieve adequate nutrition.

Dysarthria: Difficulty articulating words (speaking clearly).

Electrodiagnostic tests: A set of tests (nerve conduction study and electromyography [EMG] study) that measure the function of nerves and muscle; both together are called an "EMG test." See *nerve conduction tests* and *electromyography test* for more information.

Electromyography (EMG) test: Test performed on muscles to determine if the number of lower motor neurons going to the muscles is reduced.

El Escorial criteria: Set of criteria to aid in the clinical diagnosis of ALS.

Embryonic stem cells: Stem cells obtained after the initial divisions of a fertilized ovum.

Emotional lability: Exaggerated laughing or crying that cannot be easily controlled and without underlying joy or sadness. Also called pseudobulbar affect.

Emphysema: Disease of the lungs with damage to lung tissue.

Endoscopy: Procedure introducing a fiber-optic instrument inside the body to view an organ.

Endotracheal tube: A tube that is inserted into the mouth and extends into the trachea, allowing control of ventilation; usually placed when there is sudden respiratory failure.

Epidemiology: Study and analysis of patterns, causes, and effects of a disease from studying populations.

Equipoise: A state of balance; in drug research, assuming that a new drug is as likely to be effective as it is to be ineffective or even harmful, thereby giving the drug and the placebo an equal chance.

Estate: All assets of an individual.

Excitotoxicity: Death of a nerve cell as a result of being excited to an excessive degree.

Extensor spasm: Involuntary reflex activity with sudden straightening of the legs (or occasionally flexion of the legs at the knees) due to spasticity.

Eye-gaze technology: Device that tracks the direction of a viewer's eye gaze onto a computer screen in order to identify letters to spell out words.

Familial ALS (fALS): Genetic form of ALS thought to be due to a gene mutation passed from parent to child.

Fasciculations: Brief, spontaneous muscle twitches; associated in ALS with loss of lower motor neurons.

Fluoroscopy: X-ray study of moving body structures.

Footdrop: Condition with weakness of the muscles that control movement of the ankle, causing the foot to drag.

Forced vital capacity (FVC): Test of diaphragm muscle strength that measures how much air can be taken in and exhaled.

Frontal lobes: Portions of the brain at the front of the cerebral hemispheres.

Frontotemporal dementia (FTD): See *frontotemporal lobe dementia.*

Frontotemporal lobe dementia (FTLD): Type of dementia due to degeneration of nerve cells in the frontal and temporal lobes of the brain. Also called frontotemporal dementia.

Gastric feeding tube (G-tube): Tube placed in the stomach that allows nutrition and fluids to be delivered without the need to swallow.

Gastroenterologist: A doctor with training in gastroenterology (disorders of the digestive system). Gastroenterologists place gastric feeding tubes.

Gastrostomy: The procedure of placing a feeding tube directly in the stomach.

Gene: A segment of DNA that contains the code to make a protein.

Genetic counselor: A healthcare provider who explains and provides counseling concerning genetic disorders and tests for them.

Genetic factor: A disease that may be caused by or contributed to by one or more gene mutations.

Glial cells: Cells in the nervous system that support nerve cells.

Glutamate: An amino acid that serves as the neurotransmitter that activates upper and lower motor neurons.

Healthcare provider: Health professional with specialized training in a particular area of medicine.

Hereditary: Of a trait or a disease, able be passed on to offspring.

Hospice: Medical care during the terminal stages of an illness.

Immune system: A complex defense system in the body that recognizes invading germs and destroys them; also responsible for cleaning up cells that have died.

Invasive ventilation: Use of a breathing machine that meets all of a patient's respiratory needs.

J-tube: A tube that is similar to a gastric feeding tube (G-tube) but is placed in the jejunum (the first part of the small intestine).

Laparoscopy: Surgical procedure that uses fiber optics to visualize organs for surgery.

Laryngeal spasm: Brief situation of shortness of breath due to tightening of the vocal cords making the passage of air across the larynx difficult; frequently results in a harsh sound called stridor.

Larynx: Region of the throat that contains the vocal cords. Also known as the voice box.

Living will: Document listing what medical procedures a person would want or not want if unable to voice his or her decisions.

Locked-in: Situation where an ALS patient is aware but cannot communicate verbally or by movements because of profound weakness.

Lower motor neurons: Groups of nerve cells in the brainstem and spinal cord that send nerve fibers to muscles.

Lumbosacral spine region: The lower back where it joins the pelvis, including the bony spine (vertebrae) and the nerve roots.

Lymph system: A network of vessels that take up fluid (lymph) and transport it into the blood circulation.

Magnetic resonance imaging (MRI): A technique for imaging the brain and spinal cord using pulsed magnetic fields.

Maximum inspiratory force (MIF): See *maximum inspiratory pressure*.

Maximum inspiratory pressure (MIP): Breathing test of diaphragm muscle strength. Also called maximum inspiratory force.

Mesenchymal stem cells: Stem cells obtained from adipose (fat) tissue.

Mitochondria: Tiny structures in all cells that produce energy for all cellular functions.

Motor neuron disease (MND): General term that includes ALS, primary lateral sclerosis (PLS), progressive muscular atrophy (PMA), and progressive bulbar palsy (PBP).

Multidisciplinary ALS clinic: A medical clinic that includes a number of providers, allowing the ALS patient to be seen by practitioners of many disciplines in one visit.

Mutation: An error in the genetic code that leads to the production of an abnormal protein or no protein.

Myelopathy: Injury to the spinal cord resulting in spasticity in the legs due to damage of upper motor neuron fibers.

Nerve conduction tests: Tests performed by a neurologist to determine if there are abnormalities of sensory or motor nerves.

Nerve growth factors: Proteins initially produced during fetal development to govern nerve growth but that can also help support nerve cells that are degenerating.

Neurodegeneration: Degeneration and death of nerve cells due to a progressive disease process.

Neurologist: A doctor who specializes in diseases of the nervous system.

Neuropsychologist: A psychologist who specializes in testing cognitive (thinking) function.

Neuron: A nerve cell that connects one nerve cell to another or to muscles.

Neurotransmitter: A chemical that transmits excitation from one nerve cell to another or from a nerve cell to a muscle.

Noninvasive ventilation: Use of a breathing machine that aids a patient's respiration.

Nurse: A healthcare provider who works with the neurologist and other healthcare providers to coordinate the overall care of the patient and to communicate with the caregiver.

Occupational therapist: A healthcare professional who assesses the use of hands and arms for daily activities and makes suggestions to enhance function.

Orthopnea: Shortness of breath when lying supine (on one's back).

Orthotist: A healthcare provider who assesses which ankle braces will be most effective.

Oxidative stress: Metabolic stress within cells.

Oximetry: Measurement of the oxygen level in the blood by placing a clip on a finger or at night during sleep (nocturnal oximetry).

Palliative care: Multidisciplinary approach to caring for patients who have progressive disorders in such a way as to optimize their comfort.

Percutaneous endoscopic gastrostomy (PEG): A technique for inserting a gastric feeding tube using endoscopy.

Phrenic nerve: Lower motor nerve that goes from the spinal cord to the diaphragm.

Physical therapist: A healthcare professional who assesses the use of legs and makes suggestions to enhance mobility.

Placebo: A pill or procedure that contains no active ingredient but looks the same as an active pill or procedure.

Polysomnogram: Study where brainwaves, breathing effort, and other measures are obtained during sleep in a special sleep laboratory.

Power of attorney for financial affairs: Document that entrusts another person to make decisions about financial matters if the individual is unable to make such decisions.

Power of attorney for healthcare: Document that entrusts another person to make decisions about medical care if the individual is unable to make such decisions. Also called a power of attorney for medical affairs.

Primary care physician (PCP): Doctor who provides care for general medical problems.

Proprioceptive: Related to proprioception, the perception a person has of where his or her limbs and body are in space.

Primary lateral sclerosis (PLS): Form of motor neuron disease involving loss only of upper motor neurons.

Progressive bulbar palsy (PBP): Form of motor neuron disease involving loss only of upper motor neurons affecting speech and swallowing.

Progressive muscular atrophy (PMA): Form of motor neuron disease involving loss only of lower motor neurons.

Pseudobulbar affect (PBA): A condition frequently occurring in ALS that is characterized by easily occurring laughing and crying that is beyond the control of the patient. Also called emotional lability.

Psychiatrist: A doctor who specializes in disorders of mood.

Psychologist: A healthcare professional who evaluates disorders of thinking and mood.

Pulmonologist: A doctor who specializes in the care of breathing disorders.

Radiologically inserted gastrostomy (RIG): A technique for inserting a gastric feeding tube using fluoroscopy.

Rapid eye movement (REM) sleep: Phase of sleep where all muscles are paralyzed except for the diaphragm and the muscles that move the eyes.

Respiratory therapist: A healthcare professional who assesses difficulties with breathing and makes suggestions for interventions to enhance breathing.

Respite: A rest or break from caring for a patient.

Response shift: A shift in a person's perception of what makes for a satisfactory quality of life. Such shifts are a normal part of aging and also occur in the setting of a disability such as ALS.

Resuscitate: To revive a patient from apparent death.

Rilutek: See *riluzole*.

Riluzole: Only FDA-approved drug (brand name Rilutek) that slows the progression of ALS to even a modest degree.

Risk factor: A characteristic or exposure that increases an individual's risk of developing a disease.

Sclerosis: Pathology term for hardening. In ALS, hardening in the spinal cord due to scar tissue after loss of upper motor neuron fibers.

Selective serotonin reuptake inhibitors (SSRIs): A class of mood-elevating drugs.

Social worker: A healthcare provider who assists with social services (such as insurance and disability issues) and serves as a counselor.

Spastic: Characterized by stiffness of speech or of arm or leg movement (spasticity) due in ALS to loss of upper motor neurons.

Speech-language pathologist: A healthcare provider who evaluates swallowing and speech disorders and makes suggestions to enhance function.

Spinal cord: Portion of the nervous system that lies within the bony vertebrae and connects to the brainstem.

Split hand syndrome: Pattern of hand muscle weakness frequently observed in ALS in which the thumb side of the hand is affected before the little-finger side.

Sporadic ALS (sALS): ALS in a person who has no other family members with the disease.

Support group: Gathering of patients and caregivers to share information and discuss issues.

Synapse: Microscopic space between two nerves where neurotransmitters from one nerve cross and activate the second nerve.

Temporal lobes: Portions of the cerebral hemispheres that lie at the sides of the brain.

Trachea: The open tube between the throat and the lungs. Also known as the windpipe.

Tracheal tube: A metal or plastic tube surgically placed in the trachea to allow connection to a ventilator.

Tracheostomy: A surgical procedure creating an opening in the trachea; also, the opening so made.

Trust: A financial arrangement whereby one individual (the trustor) places assets in the care of another individual (the trustee), who is designated to administer those assets according to terms specified in the trust agreement.

Trustee: Person given powers to act on behalf of another person in specific situations.

Upper motor neurons: Nerve cells in the motor cortex of the brain that connect to lower motor neurons.

Urgency: The sudden need to urinate or move one's bowels.

Will: Set of written instructions for how an individual wishes to have his or her possessions and money distributed upon his or her death.

X-linked inheritance: Inheritance pattern where in order for a disease to develop, one copy of the abnormal gene (mutation) needs to be present on an X chromosome and the other chromosome must be a Y chromosome. Thus only males can have the disease. Females can be carriers of the mutation but cannot have the disease.

About the American Academy of Neurology

The American Academy of Neurology is the world's largest association of neurologists and neuroscience professionals, with 30,000 members. The AAN is dedicated to promoting the highest quality patient-centered neurologic care. A neurologist is a doctor with specialized training in diagnosing, treating, and managing disorders of the brain and nervous system such as Alzheimer's disease, stroke, migraine, multiple sclerosis, concussion, Parkinson's disease, and epilepsy.

For more information about the American Academy of Neurology, visit *AAN.com* or find us on Facebook, Twitter, LinkedIn, and YouTube.

To sign up for a free subscription to *Neurology Now®*, the Academy's magazine for patients and caregivers, visit *NeurologyNow.com*.

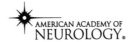

About the American Brain Foundation

The American Brain Foundation is a national foundation whose mission is to bring researchers and donors together to defeat brain disease. Through cross-cutting innovative research, the American Brain Foundation is making investments in the best and brightest minds in the world to identify treatments, prevention methods, and cures for brain disease.

Learn more at *AmericanBrainFoundation.org* or find the Foundation on Facebook, Twitter, Google+, and YouTube.

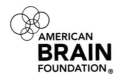

INDEX

References to figures and tables are denoted by an italicized *f* and *t*.